The Germ of Laziness

# THE GERM

## OF

# LAZINESS

## Rockefeller Philanthropy
## and Public Health
## in the New South

John Ettling

Harvard University Press
Cambridge, Massachusetts
and London, England
1981

Publication of this book has been aided by a grant from the Andrew W.
Mellon Foundation

**Library of Congress Cataloging in Publication Data**

Ettling, John, 1944–
　　The germ of laziness.

　　Includes bibliographical references and index.
　　1. Hookworm　disease – Southern　States – Prevention – History –
20th century.　　2. Rockefeller Sanitary Commission for the Eradica-
tion of Hookworm Disease – History.　　3. Public health – Southern
States – History – 20th century.
I. Title.
RA644.H65E88　　　　362.1'969654　　　81-4174
ISBN 0-674-34990-3　　　　　　AACR2

For my parents,

Albert J. Ettling
Emily Tucker Ettling

# Preface

In 1909, with the progressive movement at flood tide, John D. Rockefeller, himself the object of so much reformist wrath, announced the creation of a comparatively modest and short-lived organization to confront a disease few people had heard of. Launched with a $1 million grant, the Rockefeller Sanitary Commission for the Eradication of Hookworm Disease was certainly not Rockefeller's first or his largest philanthropic enterprise. Measured against the impressive dimensions of the University of Chicago or the General Education Board, the Sanitary Commission was puny indeed. And unlike Rockefeller's loftier benefactions, the Sanitary Commission was never intended to endure. In fact, after a five-year campaign in eleven Southern states, the Sanitary Commission passed out of existence, its remaining objectives and unexpended funds assimilated into the more recently created and much more ambitious Rockefeller Foundation.

In view of its limited scope and duration, why go to such lengths to study the Sanitary Commission? In the first place, its creation in 1909 marks the convergence of two separate tributaries of American philanthropy: scientific medicine and public education. Each had benefited from Rockefeller's and other men's benevolence in the past. But the special imperatives of the campaign against hookworm disease brought about a marriage of the two, required by the nature of hookworm disease and the fact that so few people in the early twentieth century knew of its existence. The Sanitary Commission also contributed more to the growth of the American public health movement and to the improvement of the quality of life in the rural South than its small endowment and brief tenure might at first glance imply. In the course of its five-year life, the Sanitary Commission awakened Southerners to the widespread presence and detrimental impact of this disease in their midst; it underwrote the first important steps toward amelioration; it energized the moribund Southern state boards of health; and it served as the immediate prototype for the far more extensive early overseas work of the Rockefeller Foundation.

The story of the Commission unfolds against the larger backdrop of American reform in the early twentieth century. It is a compelling story in its own right, self-contained, with an unusual degree of dramatic unity. Scaled down without distortion to fit the proportions of the Sanitary Commission and crowded into this little diorama of scenes from Southern country life is a miniature Augean stable of progressive chores. Within the context of the hookworm campaign, in large part *because* its goals were so limited and sharply defined, it is possible to consider one unified set of working solutions to problems that bedeviled other, more far-flung reformers in different fields. In order to carry out its assignments, the Sanitary Commission had to forge ad hoc relationships between North and South, between city and countryside, between private wealth and public agencies, between the expert and the mass of ordinary citizens.

A small but strategically important bivouac on the march toward the conquest of dread disease and a laboratory for progressive era experimentation: were the Sanitary Commission nothing more than this it might still command the attention of scholars. But a study of the Sanitary Commission's personnel and institutional predecessors also reveals oddly shaped pieces that seem to fit larger historical puzzles. These pieces make little sense unless one examines the lives of the men who ran the Commission. No one connected with the Commission sprang to life in 1909, fully grown and fully armed to do battle with the hookworm. Led by Frederick T. Gates, the architect of Rockefeller's early charitable programs, the handful of men who financed, organized, and directed the daily activities of the Sanitary Commission came to their tasks long after they had already become well established in their respective fields. A scientist, a plutocrat, a former minister, a professor of philosophy, a journalist: collectively they brought a wealth of diverse experience to bear on their mutual enterprise. Their careers had traced separate arcs before converging on the Sanitary Commission, but years earlier those careers had departed from a common point. All of the principal actors in the story of the Sanitary Commission had grown up on farms or in small towns. Evangelical religion had been the dominant shaping force in their early lives. Most of them sincerely believed that they had shed the religious superstitions of their childhoods somewhere along the way toward becoming twentieth-century men of affairs—professionals, city-dwellers, and reformers. Still, the evangelical habits of mind remained with them in ways which they themselves could not see, but which nevertheless caused them to act in accordance with patterns that become clear in retrospect. Their agenda for reform may have reflected their acquired enthusiasm for the insights of scientific medicine and the goals of the public health movement. Yet their emotional response to the world of the early twentieth century—a world they hoped in part of transform by the scrupulous application of scientific principles—was decidedly evangelical.

In his book *The New England Mind: From Colony to Province,* Perry Miller wrote of Cotton Mather's "curious way of backing into modernity." Like Gates two centuries later, Mather had been confronted with the problem of reconciling to his own satisfaction the "philosophical and evangelical." "Yet the charting of [Mather's] crablike progress," Miller decided, "is one of the best methods for understanding how a middle-class, empirical, enterprising society could emerge out of an aristocratic, teleological order." By the same token, the Sanitary Commission, created and administered by Gates and his colleagues, can be seen as a kind of halfway house between the evangelical, individualistic, small-town worlds of their childhoods and our own urban, scientific, bureaucratic age—some of whose familiar features they, as early directors of the Rockefeller Foundation, had a hand in shaping.

Grants from the Charles Warren Center for Studies in American History, the National Endowment for the Humanities, and the University of Houston Research Initiation Grant Program have enabled me to meet expenses that arose in the course of my research and writing.

I wish to thank Joseph W. Ernst, director, and J. William Hess, associate director, of the Rockefeller Archive Center. They and the members of their staff were of inestimable assistance on my visits to New York City and Pocantico Hills. For their guidance through the collections under their supervision, I am also indebted to the staffs of the Alderman Library at the University of Virginia, Widener and Houghton Libraries at Harvard University, Countway Library at the Harvard Medical School, the New York Public Library, Anderson Library at the University of Houston, Fondren Library at Rice University, and the Texas Medical Center Library.

Quotations from Frederick Taylor Gates's autobiography, *Chapters in My Life,* are reprinted with permission of Macmillan Publishing Co., Inc.

This study has been enriched by the contributions of teachers, colleagues, and friends. My greatest obligation is to Donald Fleming, whose gracious but unwavering insistence on precision of thought and elegance of expression has guided my work at every point in the preparation of the manuscript. Paul M. Gaston assisted my initial attempts to make sense of the material. After reading a very early draft, Eric L. McKitrick encouraged me to believe the subject worth pursuing in greater depth. John L. Thomas commented on the first two chapters, and Walter Jackson spotted mistakes in a draft of chapter four. The perceptive observations of David Herbert Donald prompted me to address weaknesses in an early draft of the book. John Z. Bowers brought his extensive knowledge of the early Rockefeller medical philanthropies to bear on a thorough reading of the manuscript in its entirety. A timely suggestion from T. H. Breen led me to consider more carefully my assumptions about the audience for which the study is intended. Robert H. Wiebe rescued me from argumentative inconsistencies and sharpened my understanding of the recent literature on progressive reform. The Harvard University Press ensured that the manuscript was given a scrupulous critical review, which brought forth several astute recommendations that I have gratefully incorporated into the final version. Aida D. Donald and Anita Safran skillfully directed the preparation of the manuscript for press.

To acknowledge that Jennifer Ettling has been my closest collaborator in the production of this book should not implicate her in its errors and infelicities, which are mine alone.

J.E.

Houston, Texas

# Contents

The Germ of Laziness

# Prologue

Much has been made in recent years of the South's entry at long last into the mainstream of American life. Two of the twentieth century's great internal migrations – of Southern blacks northward and of Northern capital southward – have worked in conjunction with air travel, mass entertainment, a national communications network, the courts, and federal regulatory agencies to reduce the sense of regional distinctiveness once symbolized by the Mason-Dixon Line. Accents persist, but little else remains to distinguish the Southerner from his counterparts at the other cardinal points on the American compass. Nowadays, Southerners even fall prey to the same illnesses that afflict people in the rest of the country. Up until well into the twentieth century, however, a curious group of regional ailments held sway in the land below the Potomac, marking it off in still another way as a country within a country. One such problem indigenous to the South was hookworm disease.

The hookworm had been a hidden feature of Southern life for almost as long as there had been a South as such. Comfortably and securely berthed in the bowels of millions of Southerners, the parasite avoided detection for centuries. Other scourges, not as self-effacing, rode roughshod across the region. If never inured to the devastating outbreaks of malaria, yellow fever, and cholera, Southerners did at least come to accept with some fatalism their sudden and deadly appearance. Like avenging angels, these awful pestilences would sweep in periodic waves over the coastal lowlands and for miles upriver, striking wherever they passed. By contrast, the hookworm wrought its destruction quietly, in measures, with none of the cataclysm that inevitably trailed in the wake of the great decimating plagues. It rarely killed its victims outright but rather left them feeling weak, listless, out-of-sorts: hence its later identification in the popular press as the "germ of laziness." Moreover, someone with hookworms, especially if he subsisted on the typical, nutritionally inadequate Southern diet, was all the more likely to succumb to any one of a number of diseases which an otherwise healthy person – one not shot full of blood-sucking parasites – might readily shake off.

Like so many other peculiarly Southern burdens, the hookworm traced its debut into the lives of generations of Southerners to the English and Dutch mariners who debarked the first shipments of African slaves in the early seventeenth century. Especially adapted to the climate and soil conditions of the South and pampered by its unsuspecting hosts, the hookworm had little trouble surviving the transplantation to the New World. It flourished for two centuries in the tidewater and piedmont areas along the South Atlantic seaboard before migrating in the early nineteenth century with the disinherited Virginians, the fortune-seekers, and their slaves across the mountains into the cotton country of the southwest.

In 1861, the hookworm went to war as a saboteur for the North. No Confederate volunteer worth his salt would have admitted it even it he had known, but the enemy within secretly softened him up for the enemy without. "Those gaunt, barefoot, whiskery scarecrows" – in Robert Penn Warren's grimly appropriate phrase[1] – never realized that the Southern soil they yielded begrudgingly to the booted, blue invaders was so riddled with hookworm larvae as virtually to guarantee that a barefoot soldier would also be a gaunt one. In the opinion of one twentieth-century historian of the South, "No one can say just how much . . . hookworm helped to sustain the Union."[2]

Between 1865 and 1910, more and more Southerners in each succeeding generation fell victim to the hookworm, until as much as 40 percent of the region's population harbored the parasite. So prevalent was hookworm infection and for so long had it been a feature on the Southern landscape that people mistook the physical appearance of its sufferers for the peculiar badge of an unfortunate economic and social class. "And, finally, as the very hallmark of the type, the whole pack of them exhibited, in varying measure, a distinct physical character – a striking lankness of frame and slackness of muscle in association with a shambling gait, a boniness and misshapeliness of head and feature, a peculiar sallow swartness, or alternatively a not less peculiar and a not less faded-out colorlessness of skin and hair."[3] These were "the original lazy men,"[4] the white trash, the Jukes, the Snopses – depraved cracker types who ate opossums and married their sisters. Popular myth held them to be a bizarre accident of breeding and natural inclination. Whatever else they might have been, many were also in fact the unwitting victims of an intestinal parasite.

The hookworm entered its victim's body unobtrusively, usually through the tender skin between the toes. In so doing, it often caused a slight irritation popularly called "ground itch" or "dew poison." Once in the bloodstream, the parasite worked its way to the lungs, where it left the vascular system and entered the alveoli before making its way up the bronchial passages into the throat. From there, it was swallowed and passed into the gastrointestinal tract. It would then fasten onto the lining of the upper part of the small intestine, where it began feasting on its host's blood. The number of worms in an infected person varied from a dozen to several thousand. Securely lodged in the bowels and supplied with a virtually limitless source of nourishment, the female adult hookworm – about half the length of a pin – would lay approximately 10,000 eggs a day directly into the gastrointestinal passageway. The encapsulated young passed out of the body with the victim's feces. If they happened to be deposited on warm, moist, sandy, or loamy soils, the eggs might hatch into larvae, closing the circle.[5]

The hookworm is unusually tenacious at all stages of its life cycle. If conditions are optimal, the larvae can live in the soil for months without finding a host. Once fastened in the intestinal lining, the adult hookworm's life expectancy is about five years. Enhanced by the primitive sanitary habits of most rural Southerners at the turn of the century and supported by the South's ideal climatic and soil conditions, the hookworm's innate durability and prolific nature explain why hookworm infection easily became, and remained, such a widespread regional affliction.

The difference between hookworm infection and hookworm disease is important, although it cannot be precisely defined. Hookworm infection occurs when the worm load and loss of blood are not heavy enough to produce the external physical manifestations of hookworm disease. Three variables determine whether a particular degree of infection is substantial enough to produce the iron-deficiency anemia associated with hookworm disease: the iron content of the host's diet, his bodily iron reserves, and the intensity and duration of the infection. Malnourished people would certainly be more susceptible to the harmful effects of hookworm infection, and a 1966 study has suggested that "a supplemental high dietary iron regimen may give rise to modest increases in hemoglobin levels in subjects with light infections." The same study also found, however, that an iron-rich diet "is usually ineffective in subjects with heavy infections."[6] An adequate diet may increase a person's resistance to the medical problems that can result from hookworm infection, but only if the infection remains light. If the same person continues to walk barefooted on contaminated ground, the number of hookworms in his intestines will invariably increase and eventually overcome his higher resistance. The 1966 study concluded that "anemia may be produced by hookworm infection, provided it is severe enough, in the face of a diet which appears adequate in every respect, including iron and protein intakes."[7]

Although their ancestors brought hookworms to North America, Southern blacks proved less susceptible to hookworm infection than Southern whites. The reasons for their higher tolerance still remain unclear. No one would argue that their diets were better or their living conditions less squalid. It has been suggested that natural selection may have played a part, since Africans had been living with hookworms for centuries. Whatever the explanation, the racial disparity in susceptibility to hookworm infection provides an ironic, if small, footnote to the history of the Southern labor system.[8]

The physical manifestations of the advanced stages of hookworm disease were striking. The following passage quotes the account of a doctor active in fighting hookworm early in the century:

Persons with hookworm disease become pale and anemic, and complain of indigestion. In children, development, both physical and mental, is retarded and an infected child is dull and backward at school. In adults the symptoms vary with the intensity of the infection. A victim may feel weak, tire easily, and have shortness of breath. Also, infected persons may crave and eat unusual things such as paper, green fruit, chalk, clay and dirt – such persons are called "dirt eaters." Their muscles become weak, causing the abdomen to become prominent and enlarged, known as "potbelly", and the shoulder blades to stick out, "angel wings."[9]

The hundreds of photographs of hookworm victims (many of whom were undoubtedly also malnourished – another possible explanation for "potbelly" and "angel wings") in the archives of the Rockefeller Foundation bear mute testimony to the accuracy of this description. In case after case, whole families or settlements were misshapen and degenerate, and had been so for generations. The "Forkemites" of Virginia made up a special clan of this sort:

Lying a few miles northeast from Emmerton in Richmond county and extending over the border into Northumberland and Westmoreland counties is a large scope of country which for generations has been inhabited by a people set apart by marked peculiarities from the people surrounding them on every side. The people are called "Forkemites," the term deriving from the fact that the nucleus of the community lies in the wide-spreading fork of a tidewater creek; and for generations the name has been a by-word. Lack of energy and thrift has brought to the Forkemites extreme poverty with the inevitable mental and moral results.[10]

Abnormal dietary preferences such as dirt-eating were long believed to be a special consequence of hookworm disease, but recent investigation has called this into question. Pica, the technical name used to describe a predilection for eating inedible substances, is in fact common among people suffering from iron-deficiency anemia. Still, no one has as yet been able to demonstrate a symptomatic relationship between the two. In 1971, an American historian suggested, on the basis of his research among Mississippi clay eaters, that pica may well be a cultural phenomenon, or habit, not necessarily stemming from a pathological condition. Be that as it may, dirt-eating was observed in association with hookworm disease in enough instances to convince investigators in the early twentieth century that a connection did exist between affliction and predisposition.[11]

Diagnosis of hookworm infection could often be made from across the room, as in the case of the Forkemites. But in less severe infections, a microscopic examination of the suspected victim's stool would give conclusive proof by ascertaining the presence or absence of eggs. The cure, developed by an Italian in the 1880s, was practically as simple as the method of diagnosis, although it entailed grave risk to the health, or even the life, of the patient if the instructions were not followed to the letter. A dose of thymol[12] followed by an Epsom salts chaser (on an empty stomach) would first jolt the worms loose from the intestinal wall and then forcibly expel them from the system. At the turn of the century, an average treatment cost about fifty cents. Prevention of reinfection proved much more difficult. First, the former hookworm victim had to be taught to wear shoes whenever he walked about outdoors. Then he had to be persuaded to overcome his reluctance to answer the call of nature in a privy rather than in the barnyard or behind the nearest bush. Finally, he had to be provided with a sanitary outhouse, one that would not serve as a festering terminal for the parasite's further proliferation.

In Europe, where hookworm disease was a relatively minor problem, it had been a recognized pathological condition since the 1840s, and its antidote a patent tool in the therapeutic arsenal of European physicians since the 1880s. In the American South, where the hookworm played havoc with both the economic and physical well-being of millions, hookworm disease went virtually unrecognized until early in the twentieth century. But as the nineteenth century wore on, more and more bright young Americans travelled to Europe for an education in medicine and the medical sciences. Sooner or later one of them was certain to see stamped in the features of his Southern countrymen the telltale outward manifestations of a disease he had heard described by his European professors.

The first to make the connection and then systematically to follow up his hunch with extensive investigations was Charles Wardell Stiles (1867-1941), a New York-born and German-trained zoologist with the Department of Agriculture's Bureau of Animal Industry. In the 1890s Stiles began preaching the existence of hookworm disease in the South, but few people took him seriously until 1908, when he was able to bend the collective ear of the men who managed John D. Rockefeller's philanthropies. For eighteen years, then, one man embodied the attack on hookworm disease. The story of the campaign to eradicate it in the South should rightfully begin with the story of Charles Wardell Stiles.

# One

# MAN'S MEDICINE, GOD'S MONEY

# Charles Wardell Stiles: From Minister's Son to Medical Scientist

Charles Wardell Stiles belonged to that generation of American scientists and social theorists which had been trained in Germany or in the new American graduate schools patterned after German universities and which had come of age in the late nineteenth century with both a vision of the well-managed society and the formal skills necessary to assist in its construction. In fact, so great a debt did American reform owe to the German experience that in 1915 the young journalist Randolph Bourne foresaw in the rising tide of anti-German sentiment following the outbreak of war in Europe the sure death of American progressivism. "To refuse the patient German science . . . the valor of the German ideals," he warned, "would simply be to expatriate ourselves from the modern world."[1]

Yet whatever the progressives had achieved in the United States had not come about through a doctrinaire application of German standards to American realities. The fortunes of reformers rose or fell on their ability to modify the German blueprint to accommodate the irregularities of the American terrain. Bourne knew this as well as anyone: "What is . . . our own progressivism," he asked, "but a German collectivism, half-heartedly grafted on a raw stock of individualist 'liberty,' . . . diluted with evangelical Christianity"?[2]

Bourne's definition of the progressive movement as a whole will serve just as readily to characterize many of the reformers themselves, men and women whose professional instincts were grafted (if not always half-heartedly than often uncertainly) onto an older individualistic and evangelical stock. Nowhere is this better illustrated than in the career of Charles Wardell Stiles, widely hailed after 1910 as the "discoverer of hookworm disease" in the United States. Without his rigorous German training, it is unlikely Stiles would have enjoyed that distinction.

Stiles was born on May 15, 1867, in Spring Valley, New York. A small farming community in the hills just west of the Hudson River, Spring Valley lay well outside the gravitational field of the metropolis downriver and off the lines of trade and communication radiating out from New York to the other cities of the Northeast. Life there, when he was growing up, followed the timeless rhythms of family farm and simple orthodoxy.

What little is known of his early life was furnished either directly or indirectly by Stiles himself, but not before he was well into his sixties.[3] He set forth for his biographers a childhood unremarkable in every respect save for its suspicious fidelity to the requirements of the minor but then flourishing literary genre that governed nineteenth-century American boyhoods. With one eye always on what was to come, he carefully gathered a collection of impressions clearly intended to project a picture of an exuberantly resourceful small-town boy, carefree and self-reliant. The architect of this reconstruction, however, never lost sight of the fact that his Tom Sawyer was destined to become Martin Arrowsmith.

Like all good dramatic monologues, Stiles's reveals much more than he either intended or possibly knew himself. During the Spanish-American War he worked closely for a time with Andrew D. White, the historian and university president then stationed in Germany as the American ambassador. Stiles would have served accuracy more faithfully had he relied less on *The Adventures of Tom Sawyer* for his autobiographical leitmotif, and more on White's *History of the Warfare of Science and Christendom*.

Both his father and paternal grandfather were Methodist ministers with rather fixed ideas regarding his proper goals and behavior. Though Spring Valley lay too far south to fall within the technical boundaries of New York's burned-over district, both men saw to it that he was brought up in the bracing atmosphere of evangelical Protestantism. Both held fond hopes, frequently expressed, that he would follow them into the ministry. Stiles, on the other hand, wanted to be a scientist. The tension produced by their clash of wills, all the more intense for want of release, marked his years at home. Though Stiles never candidly acknowledged it either at the time or later, two incidents from his youth suggest its presence, and another points to its corrosive effect.

Stiles alluded to his family's religious severity only once when he jokingly attributed his facility for languages to his father's piety. A good Christian boy, in the opinion of the two ministers, should spend his Sunday mornings in church and his Sunday afternoons in one of three ways: reading the Bible, singing hymns, or meditating in the churchyard. Faced with bleak alternatives, Stiles chose the Bible. His sense of deprivation must have been doubly keen, for the countryside around Spring Valley offered not only freedom from surveillance but also fascinating diversions for a budding naturalist. His friends might waste their time in outdoor frolicking; he would be seated in the parlor keeping company with the Prophets. Intended as an exercise in Christian duty and moral discipline, the Sunday afternoon lessons, in his hands, became an irreligious intellectual game. Over the course of innumerable Sabbaths, he mastered the Bible in French, Latin, Greek, German, and Italian. Lost somewhere in the welter of new words and constructions, the ostensible purpose of the assignments atrophied. Powerless to countermand his father's directive openly, he thoroughly subverted its intent. Stiles later offered the story as a lighthearted example of a minor triumph of irrepressible youthful high spirits over well-intentioned parental constraint. Although there is nothing patently ominous in his account, one suspects that the young Stiles was driven by something much stronger than good-natured obstinacy, if only because he was forced to keep up the charade week in and week out for as along as he lived at home.[4]

When his son was just ready to enter high school, the Reverend Stiles answered the call of a parish in Hartford, Connecticut. Perhaps in an effort to forestall the suggestion that a minister's son might not be as red-blooded as the next boy, young Stiles devoted most of his time in Hartford to mischief, athletics, and drill with the local militia. By his own account, his conduct in school was reprehensible. He pushed the limits of acceptable classroom behavior as far as he could but drew back just short of provoking a serious disciplinary reprisal. At graduation he led his class in demerits (as well as in foreign languages); one more would have meant his expulsion. Once, when he lay seriously ill with pneumonia, the high school principal dryly observed that his life was in no danger since it was preordained to end on the gallows. Had Stiles felt more at home in his father's house, he would not have needed to establish quite so vividly a separate identity outside of it, one that could not possibly be mistaken for a pallid reflection of the minister. Yet had he not been the minister's son, he might not have been given as much leeway to misbehave. The principal would have been much less likely to joke about inglorious destinies had Stiles's father kept a tavern. Through it all, he maintained good grades; everyone knew he would do well in college after he settled down. That everyone automatically assumed he would settle down and go on to college, despite his notorious high school career, ironically underscores the soundness of the perception that prompted his rebelliousness in the first place. He was, after all was said and done, still the minister's son. The more strenuously he denied his birthright with his conduct, the more surely he confirmed it.

Where would he go? He was offered an appointment at the United States Military Academy on the basis of his militia activities, but at his family's urging, he declined. Yale was ruled out when it was learned that one of his partners in devilry had decided to enroll there. His parents, still anticipating an Augustinian reversal of character, persistently clung to the hope that he would ultimately decide to become a third-generation Methodist minister. Wesleyan College, his father's alma mater, was just down the road in Middletown. Though John Wesley probably would have disowned the place had he been able to see it in the 1880s, a few of Wesleyan's sons each year still followed in her namesake's footsteps. Stiles bent once more in the wind of parental encouragement. In 1885 he followed in his father's footsteps, though he steadfastly intended to say out of Wesley's.

Ever adaptable – at least in the memory of an old man – Stiles soon tailored his spontaneous rowdyism to the prevailing collegiate fashions. He threw himself with manic abandon into the world of secret societies, undergraduate pranks, baseball, and football. A photograph taken in his freshman year shows a sturdy, proudly defiant young man in a cloth cap, with dark, heavy eyebrows and a lantern jaw. Feet apart and hands thrust in his jacket pockets, he stands with four of his cronies behind the college cannon. Though the picture does not show it, one suspects the cannon is aimed at the college chapel. Stiles looks for all the world like the leader of an Eastern European revolutionary cadre: Dink Stover as V. I. Lenin.[5]

Stiles later fondly recalled his days at Wesleyan (which gave him an honorary M.S. in 1896), but shortly into his third semester he abruptly left. He blamed an inadequate lamp for the debilitating headaches that made study impossible. Yet the other circumstances surrounding his departure and eventual recovery point suspiciously to a neurasthenic collapse, not an uncommon affliction of amibitious American young men in the nineteenth century, especially those with prominent religious fathers.[6] Since study lamps were indeed poor, the breakdowns frequently took the form of acute eyestrain and incapacitating headaches. William James, whose clinical self-absorption engendered a scrupulous, confessional honesty, could recognize the signs in himself and accept the diagnosis, but Stiles in the 1930s, following the dimly perceived contours of an American *Bildungsroman* to reconstruct his youth, was not as perspicacious or as candid as James. The drive to keep his marks high, the willful frenzy of his life outside the classroom, and the old emotional tug-of-war between his father's plans for his future and his own inclinations surely took as severe a toll of his health as the infamous study lamp.

Back in Hartford with his family, Stiles passed the time quietly hanging around the house and coaching the high school football team. An oculist fitted him with a pair of glasses, and, as quickly as they had come, the headaches vanished. But somewhere in the Hartford interlude, between trips to the gym and to the eye doctor, he and his father seriously discussed and finally resolved their conflicting expectations for his future. The son's wishes prevailed. The elder Stiles reluctantly but graciously gave up his hope of seeing his son enter the pulpit one day and bestowed instead his paternal blessing on a career in science. Restored to health and rid of the need to continue the masquerade, Stiles abandoned the idea of returning to Wesleyan. With his family's money and benediction, he sailed for Europe at the age of eighteen to learn zoology from the best teachers in the world. He would not return home until well over five years later, long after his studies were concluded.[7]

Stiles entered a stream of American students to Europe that in the 1880s had swollen to a flood. Temporarily unnerved by his sudden freedom, he moved timidly into this vast new garden of earthly delights. He wisely avoided immediate total immersion by spending his first few months abroad living in Paris with the Frères Chrétiens, a Catholic brotherhood on the Left Bank. He ventured out of his sanctuary often enough to attend lectures at the Sorbonne and the Collège de France. His proficiency in French and German eased the initial shock. After this sheltered and leisurely introduction to student life in Europe, Stiles left Paris to join a large colony of American and English students at Göttingen, the ancient walled university city in what had been, up until recently, the Kingdom of Hanover. He left no record of his work there but did recall, characteristically, that in Göttingen the Germans taught him to drink beer while he initiated them into the mysteries of American football. Not surprisingly, now that he was more than three thousand miles away from his father's parish and out from under the burden of acting like a minister's son, he comfortably resumed participation in church activities. With several other English-speaking students, he organized a congregation which he served faithfully as choir director for the rest of his stay in Göttingen.

In 1887, after almost a full year in Europe, Stiles felt ready to give himself up completely to the study of science. He knew that the faculty at the University of Berlin was held in the highest esteem by men in the medical sciences. Specialists at other universities might offer a sounder apprenticeship in a given field, but Berlin gave the best broad introduction to the sciences in the world. Stiles enrolled there and for the next two years was caught up in a full round of chemistry, zoology, botany, physics, anatomy, and physiology. He came under the academic wing of F. E. Schultze, the zoologist with whom he later served on the International Commission on Zoological Nomenclature. Hermann von Helmholtz and Wilhelm von Waldeyer-Hartz taught him physics and anatomy respectively. Helmholtz, best known for his theory of the conservation of energy, had also conducted research on the human eye and had been the first to measure successfully the rate of nervous conductivity. Waldeyer who had also achieved the status of an Influential in German science, had literally left his name on the human body: Waldeyer's tonsillar ring encircles the pharynx. The terms "neuron" and "chromosome" were his as well. The year Stiles became his student, he was called to the court of Frederick III to diagnose and treat a tumor on the Emperor's vocal cords. Although most of his important work lay in the past, in academic circles Waldeyer still enjoyed the reputation of the most vigorous and systematic lecturer on anatomy on the Continent.[8]

Perhaps the professor at Berlin who left the most lasting mark on Stiles was Emil Heinrich du Bois-Reymond, the physiologist. Helmholtz and Waldeyer also enjoyed reputations for being outspoken, but Stiles took du Bois-Reymond as his model of the scientist as advocate. The director of the splendid, recently completed Institute for Physiology on the Dorotheenstrasse, du Bois-Reymond was approaching the end of a distinguished career given over with a concentration bordering on obsession to an experimental analysis of electrophysiology. In the 1840s he had detected and explained the electrical impulses governing nerve activity. In his lectures, however, du Bois-Reymond ranged outward from his scientific base to a comprehensive theory of Western cultural history. Not one to keep to himself his ideas on problems beyond his strictly scientific competence, du Bois-Reymond was a center of controversy when Stiles knew him. His political opinions (he despised the French, except for Voltaire and Diderot), his aesthetic judgments (he found Goethe murky and *Faust* full of contradictions), his views on the limitations of research (he felt science had failed to solve any of the important riddles of the universe), and his religious beliefs (he was an obstreperous atheist) angered intellectuals, scientists, and churchmen alike. Constantly embroiled in highly publicized disputes, du Bois-Reymond was personally charming and devoted to his friends. Stiles remembered him as a brilliantly demonstrative lecturer with a flair for the dramatic. Once, to emphasize the feasibility of committing suicide by interfering with the normal physiological processes, he placed himself in so complete a trance that his nervous lecture assistant had to revive him in full view of Stiles and a class of other horrified notetakers.[9]

Stiles's classmates at the University of Berlin reflected the caliber of the faculty. Three of his friends, Richard Heymons, Max Verworn, and Friedrich Schaudinn, went on to achieve international reputations in zoology, physiology, and protozoology. Another fellow student invited him home from time to time for dinner, which enabled Stiles to enjoy an occasional relaxed conversation with the young man's father, Rudolf Virchow, the father of modern pathology.

At the end of his second year in Berlin, Stiles successfully completed the preliminary examinations for a medical degree, even though he had no intention of becoming a physician. By fulfilling the initial requirements, however, he received credit toward his real goal, a Ph.D. in medical zoology. From his general infatuation with the basic sciences, he had begun to develop a special fascination for the relatively new field of parasitology. Schultze tried to persuade him to remain in Berlin to finish his degree requirements, but Stiles found himself drawn toward Leipzig and the laboratories of Rudolf Leuckart.[10]

Karl Georg Friedrich Rudolf Leuckart, like most of Stiles's professors at the University of Berlin, had already entered the twilight of an impressive career. He had given up his own creative research when he sensed his powers beginning to wane; the death of his son in an accident, and of his daughter after a wasting illness, hastened his decline. Sixty-seven years old when Stiles first met him, Leuckart still presided over the zoological institute at Leipzig, constructed in 1880 to his specifications. His fiefdom, the center of research in helminthology—the study of parasitic worms—included several well-stocked laboratories, a museum, and a library. It acted as a magnet for practicing zoologists, who came as guest lecturers, and for promising students on the threshold of careers in the new science that Leuckart had done more than any other to establish. From Leipzig his pupils fanned out over the globe to fill chairs in zoology in Germany, England, France, Italy, Sweden, Russia, Switzerland, Japan, and the United States. Three years after Stiles joined him, more than 130 former students and colleagues contributed to the *Festschrift* published on his seventieth birthday.

Leuckart's reputation as the midwife to a new science was based on his pioneering achievements in the field. But before turning to parasitology, he had made a name in zoological taxonomy. A Nestor-like figure in the world of European science at that time, he had not always enjoyed the wholehearted approbation of his peers. Like Nestor, he still carried scars from past scientific battles, visible to the novitiates like Stiles who clustered around his throne in Leipzig.

Leuckart had begun his medical studies almost half a century earlier at the University of Göttingen, where Stiles had got his first taste of German student life. He quickly became the protégé of the zoologist Rudolf Wagner, who made him an assistant in his institute in 1845 and, after the favorable reception of his dissertation, a lecture assistant as well. From 1850 to 1869, Leuckart taught zoology at the University of Giessen, years that he would later recall as the happiest and most productive of his life. In 1869 he moved on to Leipzig. While still in Göttingen, he had developed a new basis for animal taxonomy grounded on more highly refined morphological data. Against the opposition of many of his colleagues, he divided the Metazoa into six phyla: Coelenterata and Echinodermata (his terms), Annelida, Arthropoda, Mollusca, and Vertebrata. In 1848, a year when German tempers were already short, his future associate at the University of Leipzig, Carl Ludwig, ridiculed Leuckart's new system in a review of his first book, *Über die Morphologie und die Verwandtschaftsverhältnisse der wirbellosen Tiere.* "It would have to be considered a good thing for German science," Ludwig wrote, "if this book found no readers."[11] By making it a *cause célèbre* Ludwig assured that it would find readers aplenty: it has since come to be regarded as a landmark in the history of zoology. His emphasis on the developmental approach to scientific nomenclature led Leuckart out of straight taxonomy into parasitology, a field then in its uncertain infancy. His description of the path of the common liver fluke was greeted as one of the first real breakthroughs in the new science, and his discovery of the *Trichina* worm led, with Virchow's influential assistance, to the world's first meat inspection law. That discovery threw him into another unpleasant controversy, this time a priority dispute with Friedrich Albert von Zenker. In retrospect, it seems clear that Zenker won the race in the laboratory, but that Leuckart beat his rival to the publisher. Passions aroused in this argument did not subside even after Virchow's skillful mediation brought both reports to bear on the deliberations preceding the passage of Germany's meat inspection regulations. In other phases of this work, Leuckart was so far ahead of his contemporaries – notably in his hypotheses regarding the development of the roundworm, *Ascaris*, and the tapeworm – that verification did not come until well after his death. The capstone of his professional life (and the millstone of his last years) was his monumental three-volume *Die menschlichen Parasiten und die von ihnen herrührenden Krankheiten*, which he began in 1863 but did not live to complete.[12]

To Stiles, Leuckart was "a leader in the best sense of the word."[13] The formula for good leadership, in this instance, meant setting a high standard from the outset and providing a rough guideline but then leaving the students alone to pursue their own interests. After his stern dose of prerequisites in Berlin, Stiles welcomed the freedom he found in Leipzig. He became a favorite of the aging scientist although he spent less than a year with him. Working with a more powerful microscope, Stiles discovered an error in Leuckart's description of the *Ascaris* embryo. What had been initially mistaken for a perforated tooth, he found to be the three emerging lips of the *Ascaris*. His correction was published a year later in the *Bulletin de la Société Zoologique de France*. In the spring of 1890, shortly after his twenty-third birthday, he received his doctorate in zoology.[14]

Despite the ostensible completion of his studies, Stiles was not yet ready to conclude his stay in Europe. Four years had passed since he watched the United States recede in the wake of his steamer, but if his parents had begun to resent the regular drain on their income, they did not tell him. It had taken Stiles a year in Paris and Göttingen before he was ready to begin his serious academic work; now it was to take him another year in Europe after his graduation before he was ready to return home. He left Leipzig and retraced his steps to Berlin, where a brief stint at Robert Koch's Institute only whetted his appetite for more post-doctoral research. After another very short stretch at the Austrian Zoological Station at Trieste, he brought his European education full circle by returning to Paris. He came with letters of introduction from Leuckart to the doyens of French medical research, among them Louis Pasteur and two of his associates at the Pasteur Institute—Raphael Blanchard, France's foremost parasitologist, and Elie Metchnikoff, the Russian bacteriologist then studying immunology. It was in Paris that he had taken his first halting steps out of the monastic haven of the Frères Chrétiens into the strange labyrinth of the Latin Quarter. Now he moved comfortably in the highest circles of European science. Pasteur himself asked Stiles to act as an interpreter in the clinic and later gave him a warmly inscribed photograph in appreciation for his help. But the days of his European idyll were numbered. Immediately upon his return to Paris, he had applied for a position with the United States government. He was accepted and requested to report for work on July 1, 1891. If he had fled to Europe in 1886 to recover from the emotional aftershock of a false start in life, he came home five years later in triumph.[15]

From his European instructors Stiles had obtained the best possible education in medical zoology. But he had acquired at the same time their concept of the proper role of the scientist in society. He had observed at close range the prestige and influence afforded his teachers, manifested most impressively in their grand institutes and university-based research domains. Proud men, secure in their individual seats of power, these scientists assumed in his eyes the stature of medieval princes, pursing their personal quests into the scientific mysteries wherein lay knowledge of a kind useful to the rapidly emerging technological societies that anointed their undertakings. In the spirit of *Lehrfreiheit*, they did not hesitate to go before their university communities with bold opinions on subjects in their own special fields and on politics, philosophy, religion, and art as well. They squabbled and feuded openly with each other and competed for attention and adherents. But in return for their elevation to positions of unassailable authority, they placed the resources of their little principalities at the disposal of the citizens that sustained them. In Berlin and Paris, Stiles watched as bureaucrats and state planners listened to the advice of his professors and incorporated their wisdom into government programs. To the French officials, but even more to their German counterparts, these men constituted a valuable national resource, not just in an abstract and vaguely cultural sense, but in an immediate, pragmatic one.

Stiles drew his first professional breath in an atmosphere that nurtured this symbiotic relationship between the laboratory and the community. An earlier atmosphere, in Spring Valley and Hartford, had fostered in him an incipient belief in good works and useful labor in a calling. Despite his discomfort in that pietistic world, he had carried its legacy with him when he left it behind. His European instructors had not stifled this sturdy predisposition; rather, they had refined and sharpened it, while giving it their own focus. When he returned to America, Stiles took home his professors' sense of scientific *noblesse oblige* grafted neatly onto the deeper commitment to faithful stewardship that was his Methodist inheritance. He, too, became a scientist active outside the laboratory, a passionate advocate for the public interest as he saw it. As du Bois-Reymond had taken his controversial opinions before the public, so would Stiles. If Leuckart had found it necessary to fight strenuously to gain acceptance and credit for his discoveries, so would his American protégé. Stiles knew no other way for a conscientious scientist to behave.

His battles still lay in the future, however, when he settled down in Washington, D.C., and began working as a consulting zoologist at the Bureau of Animal Industry, a branch of the Department of Agriculture. In the absence of an American equivalent of the Leipzig or Pasteur Institute, government service offered the best opportunity for an American scientist to engage in research financed by the people for their own benefit. The title "consulting zoologist" might not confer the same prestige in Washington as in Berlin, but the Bureau of Animal Industry, under Daniel E. Salmon, maintained what was for the day a large research establishment and enjoyed the generous patronage of Congress. As the laboratory arm of the Department of Agriculture, the Bureau was expected to bring the weapons of science to bear on the problems retarding farm production. Stiles, whose training made him the perfect man for the job, promptly went to work on the parasites that plagued farm animals.

He spent his first few years back in the United States striving to introduce the standards and methods of his European instructors into American microscopy and parasitology. An important collateral responsibility as the custodian of the National Museum's helminthological collection gave him the excuse he needed to systematize zoological nomenclature on this side of the Atlantic according to the morphological criteria he had learned abroad. With Dr. Albert Hassall, an associate in the Bureau and

one of the two men who had gathered the specimens for the helminthological collection, he began to prepare a bibliography of
parasitology in the form of a card catalogue, a tedious and
painstaking task that he continued to the day of his retirement
but an essential one if American scientists working in the field
were to have a commonly accepted reference point.[16]

In 1893 Stiles published an article on the adult tapeworms
found in cattle and sheep, in which he argued for the adoption of
Leuckart's emphasis on internal developmental differences,
rather than on external anatomical features, as the descriptive
basis for taxonomic classification. Other articles and two monographs—one on adult tapeworms in rabbits, the other on tapeworms in poultry—soon followed. Though still in his twenties,
Stiles was beginning to come to the attention of the American scientific community, most of whose members welcomed his efforts
to standardize zoological nomenclature. Leuckart's system required a much more sophisticated microscopic competence than
the older method. Stiles helped to recruit and train a force of full-
time microscopists for the Bureau. Henry B. Ward, reviewing
these new developments for the American Microscopic Society,
approved the "introduction of modern methods into another department of government work," and urged his readers to utilize
the helminthological card catalogue.[17]

Stiles's old associates in Europe recognized the importance of
what he was trying to do as well. In 1892 he was elected to replace Joseph Leidy, who had died the year before, as the American correspondent to the French Société de Biologie. He was also
chosen to be the United States delegate to the International Zoological Congress and journeyed to Leyden for its 1895 conference.
The French Académie de Médecine made him a foreign correspondent, and later in the decade the Zoological Society of London
asked him to become a corresponding member. When the new
five-member International Commission on Zoological Nomenclature was formed, Stiles was appointed its secretary. Though his
education was identical with that of his fellow delegates, he did
not suffer from their nationalistic jealousies. In international zoological circles, he developed a reputation as a skilled diplomat as
well as a first-rate scientist, uniquely adept at harmonizing the
conflicting proposals of the French and the Germans since he had
been known and respected for years in both countries. It was as a
peacemaker between contending factions and as a proselytizer of
modern methods that Stiles became known to zoologists in
Europe and America.[18]

The Bureau of Animal Industry did not exist primarily as a clearinghouse of information for other scientists, however, no matter how urgently its employees might recognize the need for a common code of rules. James H. Cassedy has argued that the Bureau, in this period, served two masters who were coming increasingly into conflict. Its scientists and officials had to balance the interests of the public against those of the private agricultural concerns, such as the slaughterhouses and packing plants. Although Stiles aimed much of his early work exclusively at his professional colleagues, he also conducted investigations in the mid-1890s on behalf of representatives from each of these two constituencies. Ten years before Upton Sinclair wrote *The Jungle* (1906), Stiles had surveyed conditions in country slaughterhouses and found them in many cases to be spreaders of disease. Perhaps with Leuckart's and Virchow's contributions to the German meat inspection law in mind, he called in his report for public regulation of private meat packers. "Does this sound like paternalism?" he asked. "I hardly think so. The city looks after our water supply . . . Is our meat less important than our water?"[19]

As his rhetorical question on paternalism indicates, Stiles sensed that he was moving into an area with a political dimension absent in his earlier inquiries into the tapeworms found in livestock. Human health was in no way endangered by the parasites he had studied in his first few years at the Bureau. Their sole threat was to the productivity of American agriculture, and it was a direct and obvious one, clear to farmers, scientists, and bureaucrats alike. When he opened his investigation of country slaughterhouses, however, Stiles took up an issue composed of both economic and public health considerations. Predictably, as the problem became more complicated, as its definition permitted more than one point of view, he lost the unanimous sympathy of all concerned parties. When he turned his attention to hookworm disease, questions of economics were clearly relegated to a position of secondary importance. The link between the parasite and productivity was still demonstrable, but it was no longer direct. The point at which Stiles became concerned with hookworm disease marked the beginning of his deviation from the reigning orthodoxy at the Department of Agriculture.

# 2

# The Scientist as Lone Evangelist

Like many other social evils that came to light in the progressive era, hookworm disease could not be confronted until it had first been called to the attention of a public still largely unaware of its existence. Had the hookworm, like the boll weevil or hog cholera, destroyed cash crops and livestock, the federal government might have led both the publicity and eradication campaigns. National legislators approved comparatively large budgets for the Department of Agriculture to wage war on blights and parasites that directly threatened farm production. But the hookworm struck farmers, not farm products. Even so, had the hookworm proved vulnerable to federal regulation or censorship, the government might still have sounded the alarm and led the attack. Unlike the purveyors of tainted meat or quack medicines, however, the hookworm could not be shamed, fined, enjoined or coerced into a grudging compliance with the prevailing standards of public responsibility. It would give way only to a massive and ongoing program of education and social welfare, something few people in Washington were prepared to undertake. "I cannot find any authority in the Constitution for making the Federal Government the great almoner of public charity throughout the United States," Franklin Pierce had said.[1] Twelve changes of administration later, national politicians still had not found it.

Practically by default, then, the task of enshrining the hookworm in the rogues' gallery of public enemies fell to Stiles. He had enjoyed the full attention and support of his employers in the Bureau of Animal Industry when his work conformed to their definition of the common good, but when he tried to broaden that definition to include the farmer's health as well as his economic well-being, they demurred. Although Stiles changed jobs within the federal bureaucracy, he could not really increase his leverage on public opinion. What little public health work was being done at the turn of the century fell largely within the jurisdictions of the states and municipalities. As early as 1891 Stiles had suspected the need for a campaign against hookworm disease. By 1902 he was sure of it. For the next seven years he preached its dangers. But in the curious world of progressive reform, the hookworm did not exist, despite his efforts, until the Rockefellers suddenly declared war on it. The measure of Stiles's frustrations as a publicist lies in the amount of energy and money spent by the directors of the Sanitary Commission to create the disease in the minds of the people before they could set about the business of destroying it.

Stiles first learned of hookworms and hookworm disease during his year at Leipzig. Leuckart had devoted eighteen pages of *Die menschlichen Parasiten* to a discussion and a bibliography of hookworm disease. From Leuckart and others, Stiles discovered that the hookworm had been a scourge of mankind practically from the beginning of recorded history. Hieroglyphic entries on the Ebers Papyrus (c. 1550 B.C.) described a kind of anemia characteristic of severe hookworm infestation, although it is highly improbable that the Egyptians had isolated the distinct cause of the disease. Hippocrates, about 440 B.C., mentioned a strange disorder that afflicted a few unfortunate Greeks, causing them to eat rocks and dirt, endure major intestinal disturbances, and turn yellow though no trace of jaundice could be found. The Romans, in an early application of the law of correspondences, theorized that gold gave off debilitating exhalations that brought a golden pallor to the complexions of those who mined it. Lucretius (c. 50 B.C.) and Lucan (c. 50 A.D.) blamed the miners' greedy pursuit of wealth for their wan appearance. Avicenna (981-1037) described with such precision the symptoms of Arabs afflicted with "round worms" that experts nine centuries later could easily read the hookworm's calling card. But it was not until Europeans began to colonize the New World with gangs of African slaves – a period that roughly corresponded to one of increasing interest in scientific observation – that the reports became steadier and more definite. Portuguese, French, and English settlers left accounts of epidemics, called by a variety of names,[2] which devastated the black workers. No one at the time gathered the separate reports together and analyzed them, but the few symptoms culled from all of them closely match those of acute hookworm disease.[3]

The parasites were actually found in animals long before they were identified in man. In 1782 Adolf Goeze, a German clergyman and naturalist, came across a hair-like worm in the intestine of a badger he was dissecting. He named his discovery the "Haarrundwurm" *(Ascaris criniformis),* though he suspected his worms differed from the well-known *Ascaris.* His description mentioned "two rib-like structures" which he thought resembled hooks. Another German, Froelich, in 1789, observed worms in the intestine of a fox similar to those described by Goeze. With accuracy if not much imagination he renamed them "Haakenwurm" and assigned them to a new genus, *Uncinaris,* from the Latin for "hook."[4]

In 1838 an Italian physician, Angelo Dubini, first found hookworms of an altogether different species in the body of a young Milanese woman. Dubini came across the new parasite a second time, in December 1842, while performing another autopsy. His curiosity aroused, Dubini examined one hundred bodies for the worms and found them in twenty. His account appeared in 1843 and included an elaborate physical description of the worm, which he christened *Agychylostoma* (from the Greek words for "hook" and "mouth") *duodenale* (the part of the body in which they always appeared).[5] Dubini's worms were anatomically different from those found in other mammals by Goeze and Froelich. Noting that the parasites were quite easily detected if the physician performing the autopsy knew what he was looking for, he blamed primitive procedures for the failure of medical men to notice their presence earlier.

Although he had been the first to discover hookworms in man and had published an accurate description of their appearance, Dubini did not demonstrate their pathogenic importance. He had a hunch that the worms did not benignly inhabit the bodies of their hosts, but his observations led him to conclude that the mucous membrane on the intestine looked normal, at worst "arborescent." The individuals in his study had died from a number of identifiable causes; Dubini could not cite hookworm infection for a single death, nor could he attribute any physical abnormalities unrelated to the causes of death to the presence of the worms.[6] After Dubini's discovery, other scientists quickly began to link hookworms with specific diseases. Within ten years of his article European investigators in Egypt uncovered a direct causal relationship between hookworms and chlorosis, an anemia that affected young women and gave them a greenish pallor. It had been enervating Egyptians regularly at least since the time of the Ebers Papyrus some thirty-four centuries earlier. Brazilian doctors in the 1860s drew the connection between hookworms and tropical anemia. By 1875 European physicians with a respectable grounding in parasitology and certainly all European zoologists knew about hookworms and accepted them as the cause of a severe anemia characteristically found in warmer climates. Three fellow countrymen of Dubini's, Battista Grassi and two brothers, Ernesto and Corrado Parona, published a paper in 1878 which offered a simple procedure for diagnosing hookworm infection in living people. Heretofore, physicians had seen the parasites only during autopsies. Grassi and the Paronas had discovered hookworm ova in the feces of their anemic patients. Now it was possible for anyone with a microscope to detect the disease.[7]

While Stiles read his Bible in Hartford and secretly dreamed of a career in science, an especially virulent outbreak of anemia struck the Italian laborers digging the St. Gotthard tunnel in Switzerland. A wave of concern, prompted by excited accounts in both the popular and scientific press, swept across Italy, forcing the government to appeal to the Swiss for information. Switzerland willingly cooperated since the epidemic threatened its own citizens and disrupted the construction schedule. The doctors of northern Italy who for years had read Dubini, Grassi, and the Paronas in the Milan and Turin journals, were ideally situated to study the bizarre affliction. In February 1880, using their colleagues' new diagnostic technique, they discovered hookworm ova. Within weeks, hundreds of miners were examined and found to be infected. That hookworms were present in abundance could not be denied, yet a significant number of doctors on the scene believed the anemia stemmed directly from the deplorable sanitary conditions in the workers' transient camps. Indirectly, of course, it did. But a professor of pathology at the school of veterinary medicine at the University of Turin, Edoardo Perroncito, insisted that the appearance of hookworms and the sudden epidemic of anemia were related, even though the Alps were far from the tropics. He had watched in astonishment as the first post-mortem examination performed on the body of a St. Gotthard miner revealed over 1500 worms. Perroncito could not dismiss what he considered overwhelming evidence. He began to work immediately on the problem of hookworm, and gradually won over the doubters with a series of articles, the most important of which announced a successful thymol and Epsom salts vermifuge.[8]

The work of the Italian scientists, along with dozens of references scattered through the earlier literature, was collected by August Hirsch and included in his three-volume *Handbuch der historischgeographischen Pathologie* of 1883. For Stiles and the other students of the medical sciences in the late 1880s, Hirsch was the basic reference book. Under the general heading *Anchylostomata duodenale*, Hirsch placed for the first time descriptions of anemia associated with peculiar dietary preferences reported from Puerto Rico and the American South. No North American or Caribbean author had yet recognized the parasitic cause of the anemia recounted in their reports, but Hirsch inferred the disease's presence in the Western Hemisphere from the symptoms described. His book, which devoted eleven pages to a discussion of hookworm disease was soon translated into English.[9]

From the United States in the early nineteenth century had come several reports of unusual behavior which, to the trained eye in the 1880s, looked suspiciously like signs of hookworm disease. Much later, Stiles was to track down thirteen references to dirt-, clay-, and chalk-eating in Louisiana, Georgia, Alabama, Florida, North Carolina, South Carolina, and Virginia. Several observers had speculated on the cause; one had even noticed the symptoms in connection with severe anemia. A Florida physician had claimed that for dirt-eaters in the Ft. Meade area, "[t]he common remedy is said to be whisky or cider in which nails have been steeped." Hirsch and his co-workers were aware of several of these accounts.[10]

Raphael Blanchard, one of Stiles's associates at the Pasteur Institute, restated Hirsch's hypothesis, first in an article on the St. Gotthard tunnel outbreak and later in a textbook on medical zoology. Blanchard wasted no space in his narrative pointing out that the American authors had been ignorant of hookworm disease when they connected dirt-eating and anemia, but instead he used their accounts as evidence for the existence of the disease in the United States. It mattered little that American doctors were oblivious to the parasite literally in their own backyards. "Hookworm disease has also been observed in other parts of the Americas. In the United States, Chabert and Duncan have detected it in Louisiana; Lyell in Alabama and Georgia; Heusinger and Geddings in South Carolina; Little and Letherman in Florida."[11] Blanchard, Hirsch, Perroncito—all were important and familiar names to European students of the medical sciences in the 1880s. Stiles was to discover, however, that in the United States these names meant nothing in 1891. While conducting an inventory of the helminthological collection in the National Museum shortly after he started working for the Bureau of Animal Industry, he found several specimens of hookworms taken from dogs, cattle, and sheep, but none from a human being. The collectors of the samples were not at fault. To his astonishment Stiles learned that the American doctors and scientists had not even heard of *Anchylostoma* or of hookworm disease.

At this time, he simply regarded the omission as just another of the many serious lacunae in American zoology. In his first few years at the Bureau, he was too preoccupied with what he then considered the more important assignment — persuading American zoologists to follow the same procedures and speak the same scientific language — to devote much time to hookworms. But even without his encouragement, isolated articles began to creep into the journals during the 1890s, a hopeful sign to Stiles that someone else on the North American continent had started to read Hirsch and Blanchard. A St. Louis physician, W. L. Blickhahn, published "A Case of Ankylostomiasis" in the 1893 edition of the *Medical News*. His patient, a carpenter from Westphalia, was the first hookworm victim to be definitely identified in the United States. A year later Dr. Frank Herff recounted in the *Texas Medical Journal* that he had seen hookworm sufferers in the course of his daily practice for years, dating back to the time of the Civil War, but had only recently come to learn the name and the cause of their affliction. In 1897 F. G. Möhlau reported five confirmed cases of hookworm disease in Buffalo, New York. One of Möhlau's patients was a 58-year-old Italian bricklayer who had worked on the St. Gotthard tunnel before immigrating to the United States. It was true, as Stiles observed in another context, that there were "but few men in America who [were] giving special attention to the subject of . . . parasites,"[12] a fact which made it all the more remarkable that these first few reports were trickling in from the scientific hinterlands and not from the few centers of research on the East Coast. With names like Möhlau and Blickhahn, these investigators might well have studied in Germany or at least have kept abreast of the German medical literature — St. Louis, Buffalo, and central Texas were centers of German immigration. Stiles was pleased to see the evidence mounting but still not convinced that locally trained doctors were gathering it. He decided to undertake a personal campaign to enlighten American medical men.[13]

Virtually from the moment he set foot in the United States with his new degree, Stiles found himself in demand as a part-time lecturer at the medical schools in the Washington area. In the ten or so years after he started working at the Bureau, he had almost single-handedly introduced the subject of medical zoology into their curricula. From 1892 to 1906, he regularly addressed classes at Georgetown University; from 1894 to 1902, at the

Army Medical School; in 1902, at the Navy Medical School; and from 1897, at Johns Hopkins. From his first lecture, he persistently called his students' attention to the unrecognized problem of hookworm disease in the United States. "Gentlemen, if you find cases of anemia in man in the tropics or sub-tropics, the cause of which is not clear to you, consider the possibility of hookworm disease; make a microscopic examination of the feces and look for the eggs." But before he could do much more than introduce the subject in a few lectures, Stiles was called away on another assignment for the Bureau.[14]

In early 1898 he sailed for Europe for an indefinite time on a mission for the State Department to the American embassy in Berlin. Ambassador White had urgently requested a scientific attaché to counter the unofficial German boycott of American pork. Although an official embargo had been technically lifted in 1891 under the terms of the Saratoga Agreement, Germans still shunned American pork, and individual German states proscribed it on the suspicion that it was responsible for the occasional outbreaks of trichinosis.[15] Stiles's credentials were impeccable: he spoke fluent German; he was an excellent parasitologist with a German degree and some experience with the problem of tainted meat; he was a member in good standing of several prestigious European scientific societies; he was an acquaintance and former student of the discoverer of the *Trichina*, Rudolf Leuckart (word of whose death reached Stiles shortly before he sailed); and he knew Virchow, who had lobbied for Germany's meat inspection laws. Stiles, for whom hookworm disease was still just one of many problems facing American science, welcomed the assignment. He would be re-entering a world in which he enjoyed a great deal of prestige, and at the specific request of the ambassador. The new tour of duty would also give him the opportunity to show his wife of less than a year the scenes of his old student days.[16]

Shortly before his ship reached port in Europe, the Spanish-American War broke out. To Stiles in Berlin, the hostilities only represented another complication to his negotiations with the Germans, who disapproved of the American venture into competitive empire building. From his remote vantage point he did not learn of the first major breakthrough in the pursuit of the hookworm in North America, even though he had unknowingly played a major part in it. Since the St. Gotthard tunnel epidemic eighteen years earlier, some five hundred papers on hookworm, hookworm disease, and its treatment and cure had been published, all but a handful in the European periodicals. Yet no European journal carried the news of the discovery in Puerto Rico, at least not during Stiles's stay in Berlin. Like so many other advances in medicine and public health around the turn of the century – one thinks of Reed, Gorgas, and the early public sanitation programs under Taft in the Philippines – the discovery of hookworm disease in Puerto Rico occurred when it did because the war with Spain opened the tropics to American doctors.[17]

Bailey K. Ashford (1873-1934) had heard Stiles lecture at Georgetown University and again at the Army Medical School. His father had been a surgeon in Washington, D.C., and a member of the medical school faculty at Georgetown; he was one of the doctors who had tried vainly to keep the mortally wounded Garfield alive. Young Ashford retraced his father's career up to a point, but chose the life of an army surgeon over one spent in civilian practice and teaching. He accompanied the first American troops that reached and occupied Puerto Rico, where he remained, still in uniform, after the cease-fire. He was stationed at a field hospital in Ponce, a town of about 25,000 people on the island's south coast, when a hurricane swept north through the Caribbean in August 1899 killing thousands, ruining the surrounding plantations, and driving thousands more from their homes in the hills outside of Ponce into temporary camps in the town. Before the storm struck, Ashford had already noticed the alarmingly high incidence of anemia among the hill people and the *jíbaros*, the impoverished agricultural workers on the sugar plantations. He had been appalled to learn that they considered it a normal cause of death. Suspecting malnutrition since most Puerto Rican peasants subsisted almost exclusively on sugar cane, he placed those who filled his field hospital after the hurricane on a controlled high-protein diet. When his patients continued to languish and frequently to die, he changed his prognosis to malaria. Upon studying blood samples, however, he was surprised to find something that conformed more closely to the classical picture of pernicious anemia. But who, he asked himself, had ever heard of a whole economic class dying of an epidemic of pernicious anemia? On closer inspection, the blood smears revealed an eosinophile count (eosinophiles are cells with a special affinity for the reddish dye, eosin, or acid stains in general) almost ten times higher than normal. He dimly (and incorrectly, as it happened) recalled an article in an old journal reporting the appearance of the same distinctive strawberry-like eosinophiles in great numbers during an infection of the worms that caused pork

measles. (It is much more likely that the article Ashford was trying to remember reported on an outbreak of trichinosis, not pork
measles.)

Ashford later insisted that he had completely forgotten Stiles's
lectures on hookworm disease when he decided to make a slide
from a specimen of feces. After discovering strange eggs, he
checked a manual of tropical diseases, published in England, to
discover that he had a hospital full of patients with severe
hookworm infection. Immediately, he wired the Chief Surgeon in
San Juan:

NOVEMBER 24, 1899 — HAVE THIS DAY PROVEN THE CAUSE OF MANY PER-
NICIOUS, PROGRESSIVE ANEMIAS OF THIS ISLAND TO BE DUE TO AN-
CHYLOSTOMUM DUODENALE.[18]

That Ashford could have stumbled on a disease previously
unknown to him in this roundabout manner, as he later steadfastly maintained, is difficult to believe. Stiles had addressed his
medical school on at least two occasions and had discussed
hookworm disease, its symptoms, and its treatment. If, at the
time of his discovery, Ashford had no memory of this initial introduction to the subject, he would certainly not have been the
first student to forget something emphasized by a lecturer. But
several other factors, none of which appear in his autobiography,
merit consideration when weighing his version of the story.

Ashford, whose work in Puerto Rico was prodigious and in-
novative, later came to resent bitterly the public acclaim
showered on Stiles as the "discoverer" of hookworm disease in
North America. While he watched in dismay as his own campaign
among the *jíbaros* foundered for lack of funds, he read of the
princely sum lavished on Stiles and his associates by John D.
Rockefeller to carry out the same kind of program in the South.
Therefore, when he sat down to write his memoirs shortly before
his death in 1934, he was in no mood to join in singing the praises
of Dr. Stiles. He looked back to those exciting early days in Ponce
over what must have seemed to him a desert of personal slights,
humiliations, and professional frustration. His autobiography is
crucial to a reconstruction of the early struggle against hookworm disease in America, but fortunately for the student of these
first efforts, one need not choose blindly between the differing accounts of the two rivals, written long after the events in question.
Both Ashford and Stiles rushed their findings into print just as
quickly as they could, and Ashford's articles contradict some of
his later claims in the autobiography. There is good reason to

question Ashford's memory, since just enough of his verifiable assertions prove on inspection to be inaccurate to cast suspicion on those that lie beyond confirmation.

The origins of Ashford's resentment can be traced to a priority dispute with Stiles, reminiscent in many ways of the much earlier one between Leuckart and Zenker. The account of his discovery in Ponce appeared in the April 14, 1900, issue of the *New York Journal of Medicine*. "I have the honor," he wrote, "to report upon 20 cases of the severe anemia commonly seen among the poor of this island . . . I was led to examine the faeces for the ova of *Ankylostoma duodenale,* and found them in great numbers." Though not averse in the rest of the article to using the first person singular followed by an active verb, Ashford here slipped into the passive voice more commonly found in scientific writing to obscure the source of the impulse that led him to examine the feces in the first place. The implication in his second sentence — that he knew that he was looking for when he prepared the slide — does not agree with his claim in the autobiography that he had no idea what he would see under the microscope and could not identify what he found until he consulted a manual of tropical medicine. The article went on to describe the successful treatment of the victims before concluding on this curious note: "I shall not lengthen this paper [less than four pages] by any description of a parasite so well known and so fully described by the professor of helminthology at the Army Medical School." If anything, the hookworm was completely unknown to the vast majority of the *New York Journal of Medicine*'s readers, unknown to virtually all the physicians in the country. Only the few who had read of it in foreign journals, or had seen the handful of accounts in the American periodicals, or had heard it "so fully described by the professor of helminthology at the Army Medical School" — or Georgetown, or Johns Hopkins, but nowhere else in April 1900 — might mistakenly conclude that it was well known. The professor of helminthology was Stiles.[19]

Although he omitted a physical description of the worms in his article, Ashford later claimed he had noticed something strange about them from the first. In January 1900, after he had submitted his manuscript but before it appeared in print, he stopped on his way through Washington at the Bureau of Animal Industry. He recalled taking along a bottle of his Puerto Rican hookworms, a gift for Stiles, in what he considered a gesture of high-minded professional altruism. Stiles was still out of the country, but Ashford talked to Albert Hassall and told him that the worms had no teeth. Why not describe them yourself? asked Hassall. Ashford later remembered answering: "Oh, I'm quite satisfied with having discovered the cause of the anemia in Porto Rico. I don't want to pose as a parasitologist. If there is anything funny about them, let him describe them and get the credit."[20]

Stiles did just that. He described something very funny about them, and he duly accepted the credit for both the discovery and the description. He had actually left Germany in late December 1899, and, having arrived back in Washington shortly after Ashford's visit, immediately discovered one extraordinary property of these worms: they could vanish without leaving a trace. No samples of Puerto Rican hookworms entered the helminthological collection under Stiles's supervision until November 1902, after Stiles had specifically requested a shipment. By the time he finally located Ashford's original consignment in the Army Medical Museum, long after the *New York Journal of Medicine* article had appeared, Stiles, using another sample from Texas, had already guessed the second peculiarity of Ashford's hookworms: they were not *Anchylostoma duodenale*.[21]

Dr. Allen J. Smith of Galveston had recently found eight cases of hookworm disease among the more than eighty students at the University of Texas Medical School. In 1901 he sent a sample of the worms to Stiles. Both men agreed that these new hookworms resembled *Uncinaria stenocephala*, a species found exclusively in dogs, much more than they did *Anchylostoma duodenale*. Stiles compared them with Ashford's sample in the Army Medical Museum and determined that the two batches were identical in every respect. The Old World hookworm was larger, sickle-shaped, with hooks or teeth near the mouth for fastening onto the intestinal wall. Smith's and Ashford's worms, in addition to being smaller, resembled the letter "S" and had a pair of shell-like semilunar, ventral cutting plates instead of teeth. Stiles, who had cut his own professional teeth, so to speak, on just such a distinction in Leuckart's laboratory, realized what Ashford had not; these worms were of a completely different species from those described by Dubini almost sixty years earlier.[22]

On May 1, 1902, he announced his discovery to a meeting of the American Gastroenterologic Association in Washington. Under Article 21 of the International Rules of Zoological Nomenclature—rules that Stiles knew well since he had recently helped to formulate them—he was entitled to select a scientific name for the new species. In keeping with his belief that he had identified a New World hookworm, he chose *Uncinaria americana*, and as an afterthought designed to underscore dramatically the importance of his find, he gave it a second name as well — *Necator americanus*.[23]

When he reached into his well-stocked Latin vocabulary for an appropriately bloodthirsty name, Stiles had scant proof that he had unmasked an American killer. In 1902 the record reflected only a sprinkling of cases in a handful of states. Both of his names remain in use to this day, although within three years of his announcement, a German parasitologist at the government medical school in Cairo showed that the New World species had originally held an Old World passport. Arthur Looss found Stiles's hookworms in some pygmies from the Ituri Forest region of Central Africa who had been brought to Alexandria for a music hall exhibition.[24] With the publication of his report, the migratory route of the "American" hookworm became clear. Both *Anchylostoma duodenale* and its recently discovered cousin had started out in the Eastern Hemisphere, but only one had left home to stow away undetected in the holds of sailing ships bound for the slave markets of the Caribbean, North, and South America.[25]

The trickle of reported cases was fast becoming a small rivulet. Stiles, who had located and christened the source of the stream, wanted desperately to navigate it. But his duties at the Bureau of Animal Industry encompassed a wide range of parasite-related problems in farm animals; he could not devote the bulk of his research time to one parasite, especially one that infested human beings, nor could he leave Washington on lengthy exploring expeditions into the countryside. He needed a new job with a sympathetic employer who would indulge his growing obsession. On August 16, 1902, he found one in the Hygienic Laboratory of the United States Public Health and Marine Hospital Service.

Cassedy has suggested that the growth of the national public health agency in the early years of the twentieth century reflected growing popular support for governmental involvement in the maintenance of human, as well as animal, health. No doubt this is true enough in a very general way, but the immediate catalyst was, again, the Spanish-American War. For the first time in the history of the Republic, large numbers of American soldiers and administrators spent tours of duty in the tropics, exposed to a variety of health hazards uncommon or unseen in the United States. What would the boys catch overseas; or, more to the point, what would they bring home? Stiles's new supervisor, Surgeon-General Walter Wyman, accepted the need for an investigation of hookworm disease when he offered to make Stiles his professor of zoology. He foresaw with uneasiness the possibility that troops returning from garrison duty in Cuba or Puerto Rico and from chasing Aguinaldo's guerrillas in the Philippines might bring into the country still more hookworms, perhaps of a different kind, before scientists at home had made even the most cursory survey of the indigenous infection. His fears later proved meaningless when it became clearer just how extensive the disease was in the United States. Nothing was clear in September 1902, however, when Wyman dispatched Stiles south of the Potomac, into the field, to track down the hookworm.[26]

Stiles's odyssey carried him over five hundred miles through the cities and clay regions of Virginia and North Carolina without finding anything. He decided that he had been looking in the wrong places. The European literature had mentioned that the disease especially flourished in sandy areas, and when he heard that a region in South Carolina known locally as the Haile gold mines had a soil of granite sand, he elected to carry his search there.

I found a family of 11 members, one of whom was an alleged "dirt-eater." The instant I saw these eleven persons I recalled Little's (1845) description of the dirt-eaters of Florida. A physical examination made it probable that we had before us eleven cases of uncinariasis (hookworm infection), and a specimen of feces from one of the children gave the positive diagnosis of infection with *Uncinaria americana*. There were hundreds of eggs present.

Inquiring for the largest plantation in this sand district, I was directed to a place in Kershaw County, South Carolina. There were about sixty white "hands" on this farm. Going to a field I found about twenty at work . . . A physical examination showed that they corresponded to cases of uncinariasis. A family of ten members was selected and examined microscopically and found to contain hundreds of eggs of *Uncinaria americana*. The owner of the plantation informed me that it would be a waste of my time to examine the remaining forty "hands" as they were in exactly the same condition as the twenty already examined.[27]

Stiles had struck gold of a different kind at the Haile mines and in the surrounding area. Examinations in other parts of South Carolina, Georgia, and Florida almost all corroborated this initial discovery. He returned to Washington confirmed in the conviction not only that hookworm disease did exist in the South but that it was one of the region's most common problems as well. With the haste of a man certain he has come across something genuinely important, Stiles organized his findings and put them into print. His preliminary report, published by the government on October 24, 1902, announced: "There is . . . not the slightest room for doubt that uncinariasis is one of the most important . . . diseases of . . . the South, especially on farms and plantations in sandy districts, and . . . that much of the trouble popularly attributed to 'dirt-eating' . . . and even some of the proverbial laziness of the poorer classes of the white population are . . . manifestations of uncinariasis."[28]

Three weeks later, a Georgia physician, H. F. Harris, published the results of his own independent investigation, conducted without Stiles's knowledge, but which bore out Stiles's own findings. Harris had traveled all over Georgia, no doubt crisscrossing Stiles's path, and had found several pale dirt-eaters in the northern hilly region of the state who were infected, as well as others in the southern part whose anemia had been mistakenly attributed to malaria. Although he had been looking only since the previous June, Harris had glimpsed the dimensions of the problem facing Southern doctors. "I feel no hesitation in saying that time will show that by far the greatest number of cases of anemia in Georgia, Alabama, and Florida are due not to malaria but to ankylostoma, and that this is the most common of all the serious diseases in the region. There can be no doubt that what is true as regards the states named likewise holds true for the entire South."[29] Stiles was heartened by Harris's conclusions. From all indications, his own work had just provided additional leverage to a force that seemed to be gathering a momentum of its own. If the trend continued at the same rate, medical people across the country who read the journals would sooner or later see an article on hookworm disease based on empirical evidence. American channels of medical communication were certainly adequate for conveying such a simple and compelling message.

Less than a month later, however, a journalist whom Stiles never met catapulted the issue, for a moment, out of the medical journals and into the daily press. At Wyman's request, Stiles went before the Sanitary Conference of American Republics, meeting in Washington, on December 4, 1902. Since he had no reason to suspect that this audience differed in any important respect from the others he had addressed in the past, he gave the same talk, couched in the technical language of the profession, and updated to include his and Harris's recent findings. The next afternoon, Stiles glanced indifferently at a copy of the *New York Sun* in his Washington club when his own name caught his eye. "GERM OF LAZINESS FOUND?" read the headline; "DISEASE OF THE

'CRACKER' AND OF SOME NATIONS IDENTIFIED; DR. CHARLES
WARDELL STILES, DISCOVERER OF THE HOOK WORM DISEASE,
DESCRIBES ITS CURIOUS EFFECT TO THE SANITARY CONFERENCE OF
AMERICAN REPUBLICS."[30] The article went on to state, in effect,
that Stiles had isolated the "germ" responsible for human slug-
gishness. Although this whimsical idea certainly contained a
"germ" of truth, it also made excellent copy, and the story pro-
liferated rapidly as newspapers around the country and in Great
Britain quickly picked it up. Through a reporter's imaginative
rendering of his remarks, Stiles had achieved overnight a certain
kind of minor notoriety.[31]

The industrious, thrifty, hard-headed Yankee businessman was
a secure American archetype, but just as much a part of the country's self-image and just as great a projection of the national
spirit was his direct antithesis – the village idler, the cracker-
barrel philospher. Americans were amused to read that Huck
Finn and Rip Van Winkle owed their dispositions to intestinal
parasites. The argument which stressed heredity as the source of
social ills was already in disrepute among many good progressives, but here was its opposite – the old environmental explanation – with a vengeance. Loafing, apparently, was a disease
like any other. Dozens of jokes, editorials, cartoons, and limericks
dotted the pages of newspapers and journals in mock salute to
Stiles and his extravagant claim. A facetious poem entitled "The
Microbe of Sloth," first printed in the London journal *Truth*, was
republished in several American newspapers:

> I for long had believed that, concerning my case,
>   There existed much popular haziness;
> I for years had felt sure it was grossly unfair
>   To regard as a failing my laziness;
> Now the truth has come out, thanks to good Dr. Stiles,
>   And 'tis proved how unjust a strong bias is,
> For I, if you please, for my idleness scorned,
>   Have been suffering from uncinariasis!
> Of course, I've been lazy – who wouldn't be so
>   Who has known what the "hookworm's" fell trail meant?
> Who wouldn't, I ask, who's endured all his life
>   A confounded six-syllable ailment?

Other wits, not as adept at conjuring up phrases to rhyme with
uncinariasis, relied on the editorial lampoon:

Are you troubled with "that tired feeling"? Have a settled aversion for
getting up in the morning to start a fire in the kitchen range? If you
have, folks say you are lazy, don't they? Well, they are wrong. The trouble

with you, although you may not have known it until now, is that you have uncinariasis.

Uncinariasis? Yes; it's a disease. Dr. Charles Wardell Stiles is the discoverer. He has just returned from a sojourn among the laziest people in the world, the "crackers" of the South. Lazy? We beg their pardon. Those fellows are suffering so terribly from uncinariasis that they wait for the apples to fall off their trees, and then ask somebody to pass the fruit along ... Almost any fair day you can see on the corner of Main and Second Streets whole droves of men who are in the very last stages of un-cinariasis. Day after day the poor fellows stand around, stand around, looking at other people work. At intervals they go home and eat, pro-vided the neighbors have sent in anything, but the rest of their time they put in just standing around.[32]

Several papers announced that a "cure" had been discovered. The *New York World* heralded a "Staphylococcus anti-uncinariae," the miracle drug from the laboratory of "the eminent Prof. Weissnichtwarum," brought to the attention of the world "in an article on Faulheitskur in the *Vienna Wochenschrift fur Physiologie und Psychologie.*" The antidote, according to the *World,* was "produced by cultivating to a state of absolute perfec-tion the germ of insomnia in a gelatin of agar-agar, a colorless oriental plant, stimulated with exhibitions of tincture of cap-sicum and nitroglycerine." But the discovery of the anti-hookworm drug might prove a mixed blessing.

English physicians, acting, it is understood, upon representations made by the Home Secretary and the Premier, have cabled to their profes-sional brethren in New York and Washington praying that under no cir-cumstances shall any of the anti-laziness serum be given to J. Pierpont Morgan. "He has our ships now," they pleaded, "and if he takes any of the Staphylococcus anti-uncinariae his activity will be so increased that he will seize our railroads, our mills, our banks—aye, even the crown itself and the lion on the flag."[33]

Stiles's name dropped rather quickly from the jokes and the jeering columns, although ironically, a few serious articles took him to task for resorting to sensationalism. Ashford, stationed at the time in New York, must have believed something very close to that. By Christmas, three weeks later, the whole episode had passed as the restless newspapers moved on to something new in their continual search for items to amuse their readers. Thirty-seven years later, Stiles thanked the *Sun* reporter, one Irving C. Norwood, for "an exceedingly valuable piece of work in disseminating knowledge concerning hookworm disease." He went on: "It would have taken scientific authors years of hard work to direct as much attention to this subject as Mr. Norwood did through his use of the expression 'Germ of Laziness.' Public health workers and the laity owe him a debt of gratitude."[34] Norwood's article may have brought the hookworm problem before the general public, but it did not succeed in arousing the public indignation necessary to mount a serious attack on the disease. Whether or not the brief humorous national disbelief that followed Norwood's reportorial brainstorm impeded Stiles's public relations task would be impossible to determine. No one did come forward, however, and offer to fund a campaign until well over five years after the stir in the newspapers. One may with some justification doubt that Stiles felt as expansive toward the press in 1902 as he later did. They were poking fun at something he had very recently named *Necator americanus,* and, by extension, at Stiles himself. The jokes which may have seemed puckish to Northern readers no doubt lost some of their waspish good humor when retold in a Southern drawl. Echoes of derisive Yankee laughter must have dogged Stiles's footsteps through dusty little Southern towns and drowned out his warnings in the ears of touchy farmers whose pride was greater even than their degree of hookworm infection.

The year 1902 was an important one for Stiles, a definite watershed in his career. Since his return from Europe eleven years earlier, his professional activities had been broken neatly into segments, each succeeding project a separate toehold higher than the last, up the rock face of the scientific establishment. Over his first decade in Washington, his contributions—to nomenclature, microscopy, meat inspection, American diplomacy, and now medicine—had been considerable. While he worked at other things, each year added its greater weight of evidence to the steadily mounting case against hookworm disease. Then, in an incandescent burst of seven months, he had identified a new species in his laboratory, changed jobs in order to devote more time to his discovery, found the disease associated with it in scores of living Americans, and seen his story emblazoned (facetiously) on front pages of newspapers across the country. His career up to this point had been made up of a series of well-charted, successful enterprises. Despite the odd twist provided by Norwood's article, he had no reason to believe the trend would not continue.

The next seven years would bring a radical departure from this early course. Surgeon-General Wyman, his first important convert, let him wander freely back and forth across the South, talking hookworm to those who would listen and dispensing cures to those who would try. The years, which up until then had formed discrete blocks in an orderly sequence, dissolved into a blur of train schedules, hotel rooms, rented shays, one-room schools, and country churches—all seen dimly through the flickering light cast by his magic lantern. His peregrinations resembled nothing so much as a Pilgrim's Progress through turn-of-the-century America, where the very word "progress" was coming to assume a new national definition. Although his record of success was spotty, his failures merit special scrutiny since they illuminate, at least as well as his victories, some of the less obvious features of the progressive landscape through which he passed. Before finally stumbling on the Delectable Mountains of Rockefeller money, Stiles had first to pass through several darker regions on the map of American progressivism—among them the Vale of Residual Delicacy, the Desert of Nascent Professionalism, and the Swamp of Short-Sighted Reform.

Together Stiles and Wyman had worked out a two-part approach to their campaign against hookworm disease. One line of attack concentrated on improving rural sanitary conditions. Looss in Egypt had recently discovered that hookworms entered the body through the skin, most commonly through the tender area between the toes,[35] so Stiles began to stress the importance of well-constructed privies (and a good pair of shoes) in reducing the incidence of infection. In doing so, he trampled on very delicate sensibilities. Privies were malodorous, unpleasant places to be avoided. Avoidance was not difficult, since by his own conservative estimate eighty percent of the South's rural churches and schools did not have one. The percentage of farmhouses boasting an outhouse was even smaller. If one avoided using privies one avoided even more assiduously any discussion of them, especially in the presence of women and children. In an age when legs were still referred to as "limbs" in many circles, outhouses and what transpired in them were certainly not subjects that came up in polite conversation. Stiles recalled that after an address in a country school, he was approached by the local sheriff who nervously offered his services as a bodyguard until Stiles could make it safely past the outraged townspeople and out of the county. He was urgently advised to leave another town as soon as possible lest he be driven out on a rail. His requests for samples of bowel movements frequently provoked the same reaction. On several occasions, he hastily retracted his question at the stern suggestion of an incensed farmer staring at him along the barrel of a shotgun.[36]

Rural Southerners were not the only ones regard his favorite subject as a breach of good taste. When Stiles wrote up his conclusions following his first trip into the South, he included a section on sanitary privies. The manuscript came back from the government editors with an indignant demand that he excise this offensive portion. They had found it "exceedingly undignified, even disgusting," without a "place in a scientific article on public health."[37] Editors no doubt shared a sense of decorum with mountaineers, but they did not carry rifles. Stiles persuaded them that, with regard to hookworm disease at least, a good privy was the very *sine qua non* of health. With Wyman's help, he saw through the press several articles and bulletins on the safe disposal of human waste. The Department of Agriculture distributed some 35,000 copies of one to Southern farmers on its mailing lists. So identified with this cause did Stiles become among his peers that Harvey W. Wiley, the Department of Agriculture chemist who led the fight for the first pure food and drug legislation, dubbed him "Herr Geheimrath"–the Privy Councillor.[38]

The second important line of attack identified by Wyman and Stiles could not be pursued from the Government Printing Office. Getting the word to the people and offering treatment called for his active presence in the field, lecturing before local groups of citizens and doctors and dispensing cures. County medical societies, where they existed, offered to let him speak, although it often took a letter of introduction from Wyman to gain an invitation. No one in the Public Health Service knew as much about hookworm disease as Stiles, certainly, and Wyman could not release more than one officer to work on the campaign without specific authorization from his reluctant superiors in the Treasury Department. But no one was less suited temperamentally to charm local physicians than Stiles. Virtually from the very beginning he encountered opposition. After his first lecture at Johns Hopkins, William Osler, on the faculty of the medical school and one of the best known names in American medicine, vigorously disagreed. How could a disease, Osler asked, so widespread and so easily detected have eluded American doctors? This alone, in his opinion, constituted *prima facie* evidence that Stiles was wrong. Ironically, Osler had recently published a textbook with an important impact outside the classroom that deplored among other things the lamentable state of American medicine as a diagnostic science.[39]

Osler was a far cry from the average local physician, but he was the first and certainly the most eminent in a long line of doctors who would question Stiles's judgment. In the course of his one-man crusade, Stiles encountered the same polite, oftentimes derisive, skepticism almost everywhere he spoke. Not everyone disregarded his tidings. Stiles himself later said that most doctors were fairly receptive, and once the Rockefeller-funded effort was well under way, resistance on purely medical grounds became much more difficult. But how does one explain the early opposition of large numbers of medical people, members of the one group which should have been the first to recognize the validity of Stiles's claims, or at least willing to leave the question open pending the results of a more thorough investigation?

At first, perhaps, the message itself was strange enough to invite healthy caution, if not frank disbelief. A certain measure of inertia, it might be argued, provides a kind of protective coloration, shielding the practicing physician from the blandishments of quacks and wrong-headed colleagues. Later, as Stiles, despite his early reputation as a diplomat, came to assume the style and demeanor of an Isaiah crying in the wilderness of American medicine, his manner as much as his message alienated doctors by the score. Resistance brought out his combative instincts, and he became progressively more blunt, more tactless, as the years went by and his warnings went unheeded. "He did not make much headway as a lone evangelist,"[40] concluded one student of his early efforts. He began to question openly both the integrity and the competence of the unconvinced in his audiences, hardly the best way to win their confidence. An associate in the later hookworm work recalled: "He alienated the country doctors who should have been his main support by impugning their education and public spirit. He said they usually did more harm than good."[41] Whether they actually did more harm than good to their patients is a moot question involving social and psychological considerations at least as much as purely medical ones; that Stiles did more harm than good to his cause by insulting them is unquestionable.

Stiles's abrasiveness, important as it may be to an understanding of his later career, cannot alone explain the failure of doctors to accept what he was saying. He way, after all, telling the truth, and an easily verifiable truth at that. Complacency did not close their minds to him either, since they did turn out to listen and stayed around long enough to scoff. After all these explanations — complacency, inertia, and clashing personalities — have been thrown into the balance, there is still left a faint but lingering and unmistakable trace of professional hostility, entirely mutual in this case.

Robert H. Wiebe and others have pointed out that in this period American doctors, lawyers, architects, economists, social workers—viturally every middle-class occupational group—began to forge professional identities that overarched the more traditional ones of community and region, and to erect legal and institutional barriers around their callings. During the life of the Rockefeller campaign against the hookworm, the new societies that reflected and expressed this growing consciousness provided ideal forums for the dissemination of information, forums that would have been unavailable a generation earlier. But at the turn of the century, when Stiles alone embodied the attack on the disease, this nascent awareness of professional exclusiveness presented an obstacle he could not always surmount. Expressed in its baldest terms, Stiles did not have an M.D. degree. To many of the doctors in his audiences, he was a government man whose background was in worms and taxonomic charts. (As a North Carolina physician put it, Stiles held "an honorary degree of doctor of something else.") Unlike them, he was not called to noble service in the healing arts and, more tellingly, was not so certified. What could this laboratory man, trailing clouds of formaldehyde, tell them about their patients? His time would be better spent helping those same patients with their livestock. To some, he must have seemed a slightly comical figure, pompously and obsessively prating on about such an improbable and unseemly subject. Osler, at least, was in a position to appreciate Stiles's credentials. But Southern country doctors, whose patients actually suffered most from hookworms and to whom Stiles endlessly addressed his appeals, were not as objective. Those who still held strong regional biases would detest a Yankee "doctor of something else" who worked for the federal government. Others who had shed their sectional loyalties for professional ones might easily have dismissed him as an occupational outsider, an interloper in their sacred preserve.[42]

Stiles must surely have sensed the condescension underlying their skepticism. For his part, he undoubtedly held most of them in rather low esteem. Though he later mentioned "the favorable reaction of physicians in general," the only incident from all his lectures before county medical groups that he included in his history concerns a pair of what he pejoratively termed "backwoods physicians" who complained to a program committee that his message, if heeded, would cut into their incomes by reducing the amount of disease in the area.[43] His own strong professional pride must have made the dismissals all the more galling. He had studied with Leuckart and du Bois-Reymond, had worked with Pasteur and Koch, was on friendly terms with Virchow, while they were learning about leeches and saws in dismal places that hardly warranted the name of medical school. Had he not spent enough time lecturing in the best of them to gain a clear impression of the difference? If his associates on the International Commission on Zoological Nomenclature, who thought of him as the diplomat, would not have recognized the sarcastic and vituperative lecturer, it is probably because they would never have laid bare that facet of his personality, which emerged in response to incredulity and thinly veiled condescension. Clues to his sense of distinction, if not superiority, abound. He continued, for example, even after years of regular communication with the same administrative officer in the Rockefeller organization, a professional man himself whom Stiles knew well, to write "Professor of Zoology" in longhand just beneath his signature.[44] It is true that in Germany, where Stiles had developed his professional habits, such formalities were commonplace, but there they were accepted, even expected, by the laity. That these graduates of lowly institutions, who practiced something they loosely called medicine, ignored his tirelessly reiterated theme must have done little to increase their stature in his eyes. Surely it is no coincidence that his most enthusiastic initial converts were educators, publicists, millowners, philanthropists, and those physicians who deferred to the importance of his title, were less concerned with professional differences, and saw him only as a distinguished man of medicine.

If delicate sensibilities and professional jealousies made Stiles's work more difficult, the organized opponents of child labor, if they had had their way, would have brought it summarily to a close. Here again, as when his bluntness exasperated already fastidious natures and his sarcasm alienated already skeptical doctors, Stiles himself was partially responsible for this clash with another group which might have been expected to support him wholeheartedly. But here too other factors unrelated to his increasingly irascible personality played a definite part. The issue came to a head, amid calls for his dismissal from government service, shortly after a 1907 federal investigation into the problem of child labor, in which Stiles had taken part.

Had he had a staff of assistants in the early days of the hookworm campaign, Stiles might have been able to avoid his skirmish with the humanitarians. Since he was working by himself, common sense led him to concentrate his energies where they would reap the greatest immediate rewards. The cotton manufacturers of the Piedmont region from Virginia to Georgia, men who already considered themselves enlightened employers on the George Pullman model, readily offered him access to the villages under their control. By the middle of the first decade of the twentieth century, eighty-seven percent of cotton-mill workers were living in houses owned by the companies – the vast majority in mill villages – and an undetermined but certainly considerable number of them suffered from hookworm disease. As early as 1902, on his first trip into the South, Stiles had struck up a friendship with Dr. William Weston of Columbia, South Carolina, who had opened a cotton-mill clinic at the behest of his employers, Olympia Mills. Weston was hoping to reduce the number of man-hours lost each year to malaria, but when Stiles passed along the results of his survey, the company doctor quickly redirected his attention in the clinic to hookworm disease. The same *New York Sun* article that announced the discovery of the "germ of laziness" also reported Stiles's conviction that the health of Southern children improved dramatically when they moved from the family farm to a mill village. Although he never said so explicitly, Stiles did not go out of his way to correct the impression that the boys and girls of the South were better off under the benign wing of the millowner. He came to the attention, therefore, of the anti-child-labor forces at the same time that he came to the attention of the public at large, but the child-labor opponents, unlike the general public, did not forget him.[45]

That Stiles jumped at the opportunity to carry his work into the mill villages is certainly not hard to understand. Here, concentrated in one small area, were as many hookworm victims as might be found in a whole county full of hidden, often inaccessible farms. As the only man in the field against a powerful enemy, he needed all the allies, as well as all the shortcuts, he could find. The enthusiasm of the millowners must also have come as a welcome relief from the discouraging reception he was given in other parts of the South. The people in the town down the road might threaten and their doctors might heckle, but in the mill village, under the protection and the patronage of the manufacturer, Stiles found a docile and cooperative audience. Nor would he have to overcome or rationalize away personal scruples regarding the justice of the relationship between employer and employees, the paternalism that characterized these communities. Not one to indict out of hand the captains of industry, Stiles had already, on at least one occasion and with regard to a different matter, admonished his scientific colleagues for publicizing their theories without looking to the economic consequences: "Let us not forget that to a very great degree we owe our opportunities for research work either to direct or indirect taxes which fall upon the public or to the public spirited generosity of certain men, and we should consider the sources of support by not leaving out of consideration the economic effect which theories and hypotheses may produce."[46]

For their part, the millowners welcomed a chance to demonstrate publicly their good faith and concern for the welfare of their employees. C. Vann Woodward has argued that the animosity generated by the collision between the cotton manufacturers on the one hand, and both the child-labor activists and the union organizers on the other, was heightened by the owners' belief that they were more sympathetic to the needs of working people than any other group of businessmen and in the creative vanguard of the movement towards improved labor relations.[47]

Their form of company paternalism had been hailed by the New South boosters as an ideal way to indulge a proper concern for the welfare of the workers without resorting to a self-defeating increase in salaries—attractively low wage scales, along with a favorable tax structure and the absence of union activity, had been the lure that had coaxed the textile mills out of New England in the first place. By inviting Stiles into their villages, the owners hoped to harvest both a humanitarian and an economic dividend. In one stroke they felt they had re-emphasized their commitment to the well-being of their laborers while shoring up that part of their investment in labor which rose or fell with the health of the work force. Stiles had demonstrated to their satisfaction that much of the "cotton-mill anemia" that owner and operative alike had long accepted with resignation as an occupational hazard of Southern cotton-mill workers was due to hookworm disease.[48]

A bill introduced in the United States Senate by Benjamin R. ("Pitchfork Ben") Tillman of South Carolina, which would have channeled $25,000 through the Public Health Service to move against soil pollution, underscores the millowners' faith in Stiles. A grizzled, one-eyed veteran of the Populist wars of the 1890s, Tillman had survived, while other old Alliance men fell, by quickly making his separate peace with the large business interests of his state and by moving from the governor's mansion to the United States Senate where his tenure was not as dependent on popular support. Tillman had not been responding to the promptings of his less fortunate constituents on the farm when he proposed his legislation. Though he still struck a plowboy's pose on the national political stage, he had long since forfeited the support of the dirt farmers of South Carolina. As early as 1891, while still in his first term as governor, he had been read out of the Farmers' Alliance for "scattering the seeds of discord." Rather, his soil pollution bill had been designed to bring a measure of federal relief to his more powerful supporters who had already undertaken the program themselves. When Roosevelt's Treasury Department, where the senator from South Carolina had few friends, advised Wyman not to cooperate, Tillman lost interest, and the bill quietly died. Its short, unhappy life is of no consequence. It does prove that the cotton millowners had taken Stiles to their hearts.[49]

The critics of child labor, who grew increasingly militant as the decade wore on, had singled out Stiles's new allies as their most formidable opponents.[50] Child labor was an emotional issue that galvanized and drew together reformers from a number of parallel fields. Advocates of educational improvements pointed to the high illiteracy rates in the mill villages; Samuel Gompers of the American Federation of Labor called attention to its retarding effect on the labor movement in the South; social welfare people excoriated the long hours and the preponderance of night shifts; middle-class Southerners, who actually spearheaded the crusade, lamented the effect of child labor on the quality of life in the South and on regional traditions, quoting Jefferson Davis' admonition: "Do not grind the seed corn."[51] These disparate groups came together in 1904 to form the National Child Labor Committee under the direction of an Alabamian, Edgar Gardner Murphy. Under his guidance, the movement stepped up its assault on state legislatures and skillfully tailored its argument to appeal to Southern prejudices. What would come to pass in the South, they asked, if white children were entombed in the mills from an early age while blacks attended school and "[grew] tall in the sun?"[52]

Had Stiles been more sensitive to the nuances of public opinion he might have noticed that the tide had begun to go out on the millowners. Had he been less the public health official concerned with the number of people immediately treated and more the publicist aware of the power of dedicated pressure groups to precipitate change, he might have thrown the weight of his evidence into the balance on the side of the reformers and seen his cause taken up as their own. The hookworm did, after all, play havoc with a child's ability to learn in school, with his father's ability to work, and with the whole family's social welfare. The 1907 federal investigation, in which he was charged with a study of the health of children in the mills, gave him a second chance to get into the good graces of the reformers, or at least to neutralize their wrath. He failed to seize the opportunity. Rather than stressing the health problems he found in the mills—the bad diet, inadequate ventilation, and back-breaking hours—he gave them only passing mention. He elected to emphasize instead the slightly superior sanitary conditions—the privies, the fenced-in yards, the availability of company physicians—that the mill villages enjoyed over the farms in the narrow area of hookworm disease. He could not even forego a gratuitous slap at the reformers in his report when he mentioned that uninformed observers often mistook for children adult workers whose growth had been retarded by hookworm disease. Even the millowners themselves did not contend that their employees were really just youthful-looking dwarfs. Stiles later chortled that the child-labor opponents eventually had to acknowledge the accuracy of his facts, a good indication, if one was still needed, that he had completely missed the point of their opposition. He also complained that he was forced, at the time of the investigation, to decline an offer of $50,000 from a cotton-mill president to finance a campaign against the parasite for fear that the child-labor people would willfully misread his acceptance of the gift as the mortar in an unholy alliance between the federal government and the mill bosses.[53]

Stiles was convinced, of course, that the menace of hookworm disease far outweighed the lesser social injustices that preoccupied other reformers. Indeed, in his mind, so completely given over to the medical depredations of the parasite, the potential for treatment existing in the mill villages left the question of the justice or injustice of child labor open, if not beside the point. The awesome implications of his meticulously gathered facts should, he felt, silence the bickering between management and labor, between reformers and defenders of the status quo, as well as put to rest any possibility of a conflict of interest (especially since he was so sure of his own integrity), and weld them all into a single unit with a common purpose, in much the same way that the clear national peril in wartime obliterated domestic differences for the duration of the fight. He failed to understand that the child-labor people were just as narrowly obsessed with that evil as he was with hookworm disease. Both he and they lived in a Manichean world, but each wrestled with a different devil. Unlike Osler and his colleagues in the medical sciences who challenged him on the basis of his evidence, they cared less about his facts than about the social and political tone of his presentation. So quick to apprehend the economic consequences of a scientific theory, Stiles was curiously obtuse when it came to perceiving other consequences. If to Stiles the reformers were squandering energy and emotion on a false issue, to the opponents of child labor he was aiding and abetting in an especially insidious way—being, after all, a reformer of sorts—their particular *bête noire*. They were unable to drive him out of the Public Health Service, but the issue nevertheless continued to smolder. A year later it would burst into flame once again, to Stiles's embarrassment.

Stiles's single-minded persistence, his dogged pursuit of a goal, his stubborn belief in the righteousness of his cause, his disregard, bordering on disdain, for the outraged feelings that his methods engendered, and his failure to consider other points of view when they threatened to modify his own—in short, his fanatical dedication to a lone objective, consequences be damned—wrote the prologue of a chapter in the history of modern American medicine. In many important respects, the same characteristics had led another man from the same kind of evangelical background in rural New York to consolidate the oil business in America, thereby writing his own chapter in the history of industrial development. With the money he made in Standard Oil, John D. Rockefeller created a philanthropic empire toward which Stiles now felt himself drawn.

# 3

# Frederick T. Gates and the Business of Benevolence

Stiles never did meet John D. Rockefeller. The "discoverer of hookworm disease" and the man whose name was most closely linked with attempts to eradicate it were apparently never brought face to face. It does not seem to have occurred to Stiles to approach Rockefeller directly to enlist his support in a campaign against the hookworm. His eventual encounter with Rockefeller's philanthropic advisers, which led to the creation of the Rockefeller Sanitary Commission, came about quite by accident, without any premeditation on Stiles's part. At one point, Stiles did give serious thought to the possibility of making an overture to Andrew Carnegie, but a friend talked him out of it. "He told me," Stiles later recalled, "that Mr. Carnegie was very much opposed to thinking about suffering and disease and that when approached on his position of helping hospitals he would reply that he did not like to think about sick people but preferred to think about the more pleasant things of life, such as literature."[1]

It was only natural that in casting around for a potential sponsor to underwrite an anti-hookworm program, Stiles should first think of Andrew Carnegie. If the great steel magnate shied away from messy reminders of human mortality, he was nevertheless widely regarded at the turn of the century as the prophet and chief practitioner of the new philanthropy. It had been Carnegie, writing in the *North American Review* as far back as June 1889, who had first put his fellow millionaires on notice. "The growing disposition to tax more and more heavily large estates left at death is a cheering indication of the growth of a salutary change in public opinion," he wrote. "By taxing estates heavily at death the state marks its condemnation of the selfish millionaire's unworthy life."[2] A clause in one's will bequeathing something for public purposes was almost as reprehensible as no clause at all, since "men who leave vast sums in this way may fairly be thought men who would not have left it at all had they been able to take it with them." That a few men could amass enormous wealth was not itself, in Carnegie's view, symptomatic of an unhealthy society. On the contrary, private fortunes demonstrated the validity of the most recently discovered law of nature. Natural selection was working as it should; nineteenth-century civilization had evolved upward from primitive social arrangements according to the same imperatives that governed all life on the planet, and accumulated wealth was its finest flower. But though his bank balance might attest to his fitness in the struggle for survival, the wealthy man – that conspicuous beneficiary and living proof of one natural law – thwarted its free operation when he hoarded his money, or squandered it ostentatiously, or passed it along intact to his heirs. It was incumbent on the fittest to take the same pains and to exercise the same powers in the wise distribution of their wealth as they had in its acquisition. In this manner, "the surplus wealth of the few would become, in the very best sense, the property of the many, because administered for the common good, and this wealth, passing through the hands of the few, could be made a much more potent force for the elevation of our race than if it had been distributed in small sums to the people themselves."

How was the rich man, even if he recognized the truth in Carnegie's argument, to find his way in the world of philanthropy? Did Christianity offer a guide? Surprisingly, although he was a well-known agnostic, Carnegie thought it did. His Christianity was, however, a much qualified, updated version of the original. "The highest life is probably to be reached, not by such imitations of the life of Christ as Count Tolstoï gives us, but, while animated by Christ's spirit, by recognizing the changed conditions of this age, and adopting modes of expressing this spirit suitable to the changed conditions under which we live."

Carnegie insisted that far too much philanthropy ran counter to the best interests of society, to the point that it acted as a brake on the wheels of progress by reinforcing the congenital failings of the weak. "It were better for mankind that the millions of the rich were thrown into the sea than so spent as to encourage the slothful, the drunken, the unworthy. Of every thousand dollars spent in so called charity today, it is probable than $950 is unwisely spent." Carnegie believed, with Archimedes, that the secret to moving the planet lay in the placement of the fulcrum, not in the size of the applied force. Modernized, denatured Christian principles might offer some guidance, but so did evolutionary theory itself. "In bestowing charity, the main consideration should be to help those who will help themselves; to provide part of the means by which those who desire to improve may do so; to give those who desire to rise the aids by which they may rise; to assist, but rarely or never to do all. Neither the individual nor the race is improved by alms-giving." Even after this important restriction had been taken into account, there still existed a plethora of choices open to the willing millionaire. There were many "ladders," in Carnegie's phrase, "upon which the aspiring could rise." His own special favorites were "parks and means of recreation . . . works of art . . . and public institutions of various kinds."

If wealthy men heeded his call, Carnegie insisted they would not only facilitate the upward march of civilization but also protect their own positions by spiking the potentially explosive social issues of the day thereby leaving in place and unencumbered the economic "ladders" up which they had scrambled to their own fortunes. "Thus is the problem of Rich and Poor to be solved. The laws of accumulation will be left free; the laws of distribution free. Individualism will continue, but the millionaire will be the trustee for the poor, intrusted for a season with a great part of the increased wealth of the community, but administering it for the community far better than it could or would have done for itself."

In the event that economic incentives and flattery had not carried his point, Carnegie closed with a thundering curse on those who still chose to disregard his advice. "The man who dies leaving behind him millions of available wealth, which was his to administer during life, will pass away 'unwept, unhonored, and unsung,' no matter to what uses he leaves the dross which he cannot take with him. Of such as these the public verdict will then be: 'The man who dies thus rich dies disgraced.' "

There was nothing particularly original in what Carnegie said. To be sure, he was the first very rich man to throw down this particular gauntlet before his peers. If his provocative, sometimes arrogant language did not sufficiently underscore his argument, his lofty place in the firmament of American industry certainly did. But his opinions had been the common currency of charity reformers for at least two decades. The crucible of the Civil War, in which civilians had been pressed into service to care for hundreds of thousands of battle casualties and displaced freedmen, as well as the popular social adaptations of Darwinian biology, had given rise to what its proponents hailed as a more scientific spirit in the approach to public welfare in the United States. Civic leaders charged with overseeing the poor welcomed the triumph, in Robert Bremner's phrase, of the head over the heart. "Philanthropology," the science of giving, was rapidly gaining acceptance as a special discipline with funadamental principles and natural laws like any other. Carnegie's voice may have carried farther than that of any other philanthropist or charity reformer of the period, but it spoke lines familiar to them all.[3]

The wealthiest of the select group of American industrialists toward whom Carnegie directed his challenge, heard the message. In a congratulatory note to Carnegie (who privately referred to him as "Wreckafellow"), the normally taciturn and withdrawn John D. Rockefeller fairly poured forth his fervent approval. "I would that more men of wealth were doing as you are doing with your money, but, be assured, your example will bear fruits, and the time will come when men of wealth will more generally be willing to use it for the good of others."[4]

Rockefeller had good reason to applaud Carnegie's sentiments, for at the time the *North American Review* articles appeared, few men in their position had given much thought to philanthropy. Of course, few men were in their position. Rockefeller and Carnegie were invariably linked in the public mind, placed alone together at the summit of the American free enterprise system—masters of the two new industries, oil and steel, that epitomized the nation's economic surge after the Civil War. America's two fittest industrialists also possesssed, it seemed, a shared sense of responsibility to the society that had spawned them. In fact, however, Rockefeller, whose record of giving was practically as old as his career of accumulating, had not needed the stimulus of Carnegie's warning. His professed guiding principle, borrowed from John Wesley, regarding the apparent ambivalence of earning money only to give it away, was that "A man should make all he can and give all he can"—simultaneously, not sequentially. Suggestions were made in his lifetime that his propensity for giving developed only after he became a rich man, out of a sense of guilt stemming from the ruthless methods employed in the accumulation of his fortune. His conventional Baptist piety was well known, and many felt that all his benefactions were just part of an attempt to construct a large enough needle so that even he might pass safely through its eye into heaven. Others saw his philanthropies as a public relations campaign to shore up his sagging public image. These interpretations were bolstered by the way his career broke neatly into two parts. Until the founding of the University of Chicago, he had systematically put together Standard Oil; after 1891, he gradually withdrew from its daily affairs and let his name be linked more and more with his large philanthropic donations. Yet all his biographers—even the most hostile—have located his impulse to give in his early youth, in his strong religious background which stressed charity as a manifestation of good works. The size of the donations increased as his business affairs prospered, and they became large enough to claim public attention only after Standard Oil had already reached into the daily lives of millions of people. One month before he read Carnegie's article, he had pledged his first large gift, $600,000 (out of an eventual $10 million) to the new University of Chicago. But the celebrated Ledger A, not the creation of a latter-day public relations expert but the careful record of disbursements from the sixteen-year-old Rockefeller's first paychecks, contains several entries for charitable purposes, most of them with explicit religious overtones.[5]

If Rockefeller differed from Carnegie slightly in this regard, he diverged widely from him in another. The oil magnate was the closest approximation his times produced to a Calvinist merchant. Ironically, since he was probably the most successful industrial swashbuckler of them all, he was always something of a curious anachronism among his peers. At the Great Barbecue, even though his seat was at the head of the table, Rockefeller was the skeleton at the feast. "Most Americans when they accumulate money climb the golden spires of the nearest Episcopal Church," observed H. L. Mencken. "But the Rockefellers cling to the primeval rain-god of the American hinterland and show no signs of being ashamed of him."[6] Indeed, far from exhibiting manifestations of discomfort or embarassment, Rockefeller steadfastly persisted in his primitive and unfashionable faith until, six weeks shy of his ninety-eighth birthday, he was finally gathered to the bosom of his rain-god. He had been brought up a strict Baptist in rural New York's burned-over district in the era of the great revivals, and the stern Protestant example of his mother would remain the dominant influence on his life. For him, the old ways were always the best ways, even though his unprecedented success carried him far away from the rural atmosphere in which those ways had always thrived. As he approached the edge of American business experience and pushed beyond, he entered a realm where the only reference points were the internal ones carried with him from his youth.

"God gave me my money," he announced abruptly to a startled

interviewer in 1905, and an incredulous public marvelled at his perversity. No one could imagine Carnegie, who reputedly drew his intellectual nourishment from the writings of his friend Herbert Spencer, saying such a preposterous thing. But the Boston merchant who in 1651 wrote in his Will, "It is the Lord out of His free bounty that gives us our estates,"[7] would have understood Rockefeller and agreed with him. Rockefeller's attorney in the 1880s, Samuel C. T. Dodd, had reached far back into English common law to come up with the concept of the trust, but his choice of legal definitions must have struck his employer as particularly apt, since it precisely expressed his own attitude toward the fortune he had accumulated. Rockefeller believed that he abided by the Protestant imperative to provide useful labor in a socially beneficial calling. Although the amassing of wealth might serve as a convenient yardstick for measuring success in his calling, Rockefeller could not have admitted publicly, even if he felt it, that the acquisitive instinct had predominated in his choice of careers. For him, "the zest of the work is maintained by something far better than the mere accumulation of money." But the diligent laborer whose useful service was an end in itself would nevertheless prosper and gain control over a greater share of the world's material goods if the Lord smiled on his undertakings. As a good Protestant merchant, Rockefeller claimed that he had entered business to create new wealth and to consolidate old, for the greater benefit of the society at large, through the careful stewardship of the resources that came his way in the steady pursuit of his calling. He admonished young men starting out in business that "the man will be most successful who confers the greatest service on the world."[8]

In Rockefeller's earliest experiences, the separate urges to acquire and to husband were brought together in a graphic way. From an early age and by his own parents, he was given a vivid and ongoing object lesson in one way to harness the contending impulses. All the familiar details of his youth need not be reiterated here. Certain things from his childhood do, however, illuminate his introduction to the terms of the devout merchant's dilemma, while others illustrate the solution to it which he worked out for himself.

Each of his parents embodied one side of the old Protestant balance. Shrewd, gregarious, and good-naturedly dishonest, William Avery Rockefeller forsook the drudgery of wresting a living from the soil to chase the easy dollar as a small-time entrepreneur and mountebank. His neighbors, who knew him as "Big Bill," marked his mysterious disappearances for months at a time and his equally abrupt homecomings, pockets bulging with money. To the Iroquois, who bought his patent medicines, he seemed blessed with supernatural powers, since when he visited their villages he pretended to be deaf and dumb. The unfortunates who crowded into his wagon at camp meetings in the hope that his twenty-five-dollar consultation would cure them after their faith alone had proven therapeutically insufficient, called him "Doc" Rockefeller. "Dr. William Rockefeller, the Celebrated Cancer Specialist, Here for One Day Only," read one of his handbills. "All Cases of Cancer Cured unless too far gone and then they can be greatly benefited." Eventually forced out of New York by a combination of scandalous circumstances, he took his family to Ohio, where he first appeared in the Cleveland directory as an "herbal Doctor."[9]

By marked contrast, Eliza Davison Rockefeller was the worthy descendant of her Scottish-Calvinist forebears. As strict as her husband was lax, orderly as he was erratic, disciplined as he was impulsive, she inherited in his absences the responsibility of raising five children and making a living from the family farm, often with little or no money between his sporadic and disruptive visits. As the oldest son, John assumed a disproportionately large share of her burden from the time he was old enough to work the farm. Perhaps he also shared her fascination with his father's peripatetic irresponsibility, its pattern faintly echoing the Christian rhythms of sin and repentence. Neither mother nor son ever repudiated the "Doctor," even after the circumstances of young Rockefeller's later success placed them well beyond any dependence on him. For Eliza Rockefeller, both fundamentalist religion and rude necessity had made virtues of careful organization, economy, and the prudent management of meager resources. The conditions of her married life conspired to lift the Calvinist injunction regarding the stewardship of wealth to the level of a categorical imperative. Scarcity required efficiency; unpredictability necessitated careful planning. Although he never apparently made the connection, John D. Rockefeller, when he later stressed the importance of conservative fiscal practices as the only way to weather the lean years of the boom-and-bust American business cycle, might well have been describing his mother's role in the family fifty years earlier.[10]

If, then, he had learned from his father that one must not truckle to other men's consciences if one's own did not stir, and that one must be bold to make money, he took from his mother

her firm belief that with its acquisition – always problematic, never certain – came the Christian and very practical duty to spend it wisely and well. The common perception – a fear, really – informing both their attitudes was that there was never enough. "Willful waste makes woeful want," his mother had warned. Rockefeller was to make her prim aphorism the keystone of the philosophical arch that vaulted and joined his two separate careers. The "Standard Oil Gang" – Flagler, Archbold, Rogers, and Pratt – would eventually take his father's attitude in helping him to reduce waste in the process of making all the money they could. Gates, Buttrick, and his own son would echo Eliza Rockefeller in their advice to give it away as efficiently as possible. But all their efforts, no matter how wise or how diligent, would still necessarily fall short. After the modest needs of one's own family had been met, the doctrine of stewardship mandated the reinvestment of surplus wealth back into society in the performance of good works "with as much application of mind," in Cotton Mather's phrase, "as wicked men employ in doing evil."[11] Here again, however, sound stewardship of the fabulous profits from Standard Oil could only partially alleviate human suffering or satisfy human need, just as man's efforts were doomed to fall short of achieving personal salvation or man's intelligence of apprehending the Calvinist God. "We must always remember that there is not enough money for the work of human uplift and there never can be," Rockefeller wrote years later. "How vitally important it is therefore, that the expenditure should go as far as possible and be used with the greatest intelligence . . . I have always indulged the hope that during my life I should be able to help establish efficiency in giving so that wealth may be of greater use to the present and future generations."[12]

From his Spencerian vantage point Carnegie might carefully survey the field of his philanthropies for fear that someone, somewhere, was getting something he did not deserve. Rockefeller cared less about the worthiness of the recipient than about the size of the return on his investment in a world where the largest dividends would always be inadequate. The fact that both men imbued the worthy recipient with much of the same personal characteristics should not obscure this basic difference in their approaches to philanthropy.

By the time he read Carnegie's essay, then, Rockefeller was already deeply committed to a program of giving. As yet, however, his charitable contributions, though substantial, lacked coordination. Standard Oil was already the very soul of efficiency and

Byzantine complexity, a labyrinth of some forty companies representing the largest and most sophisticated agglomeration of capital in the history of business. Ida Tarbell, no friend of Standard Oil, described it in language that might have been lifted from an evangelist's sermon on the presence of God in His creation: "You can argue its existence from its effect, but you can't prove it."[13] By comparison Rockefeller's charities were random, ad hoc, and simple-minded. He did not have the time to organize and head a judicious and well-run venture in financial altruism and simultaneously to direct his industrial empire. Truth to tell, he also lost that competitive spark that kindled his interest in business affairs whenever his mind turned to his benefactions. He certainly enjoyed thinking and talking about them. Warm satisfaction derived from the contemplation of a godly work done thoroughly and well was pleasurable in its own right, no doubt, but its delicate and subtle flavor was lost on the palate when taken in the same draught with the headier and more powerful brew of aggressive competition and empire-building. The time had come, therefore, for Rockefeller to hire someone to take over and advise him in matters concerning the Rockefeller philanthropies. The kind of man he was looking for, in addition to possessing a sound business sense, would have to adhere to his philosophy of giving, predicated on his abhorrence of waste and dedicated to his goal of realizing the greatest possible return on the money invested. Two decades of personally assaying the merits of the numerous pleas for assistance put to his office had forced him to codify his vague fear that there was not enough money to do God's work on earth. Four criteria comprised that code.

First, his money should be given, whenever possible, to a work already sufficiently well organized to be of proven efficiency and usefulness. Second, it should, if feasible, be given on conditional terms, so as to stimulate gifts from others. In the third place, it should be used to foster in the beneficiary a spirit of self-help, not of dependence. Finally, the activity aided should in general be of a continuing character, promising to remain vigorous after the aid had been discontinued.[14]

These principles were adopted and systematically applied to all petitions addressed to the Rockefeller office by the man selected to manage the philanthropies. Frederick Taylor Gates (1853–1929) was the executive secretary of the National Baptist Education Society when, in 1888, he first approached Rockefeller with a request for funds to lay the groundwork for a new Baptist college in the Midwest. In the course of the next three years, the two men corresponded frequently and met on occasion to discuss its financial situation. Gates felt self-conscious and uncomfortable in their early encounters under what he considered to be Rockefeller's silent scrutiny, but Rockefeller was impressed by the combination of evangelical fervor and practical business sense he found in Gates. In March 1891, under pressure from his doctor to dispense with as many cares as possible, Rockefeller asked Gates to assume the general management of his philanthropies:

I am in trouble, Mr. Gates. The pressure of these appeals for gifts has become too great for endurance. I haven't the time or the strength, with all my heavy business responsibilities, to deal with these demands properly. I am so constituted as to be unable to give away money with any satisfaction until I have made the most careful inquiry as to the worthiness of the cause. These investigations are now taking more of my time and energy than the Standard Oil itself. Either I must shift part of the burden, or stop giving entirely. And I cannot do the latter . . . I must have a helper. I have been watching you. I think you are the man.[15]

Gates accepted at once, and in September 1891 moved into his new office in the Temple Court Building on Nassau Street.

In selecting Gates, Rockefeller was not looking for, nor did he get, a self-effacing factotum. Fiery, mercurial, and independent, Gates did not hide his feelings behind a screen of deference. "Your fortune is rolling up," he thundered, "rolling up like an avalanche! You must distribute it faster than it grows! If you do not, it will crush you and your children and your children's children!"[16] Rockefeller had better reason to believe that he might be crushed to death by the weight, not of his fortune, but of the solicitations for money with which he was constantly beset. Gates quickly came to learn that his employer was literally a man besieged. "Neither in the privacy of his home nor at his table, nor in the aisles of his church, nor on his trips to and from his office, nor during his business hours, nor anywhere else, was Mr. Rockefeller secure from insistent appeal. Nor if asked to write were solicitors willing to do so. If in New York, they demanded personal interviews. Mr. Rockefeller was constantly hunted, stalked, and hounded almost like a wild animal."[17]

Although he was unaware when he took the job of the eventual scope of its operations, Gates did recognize from the outset the need for central coordination if even its modest possibilities were to be realized. A minimal amount of organization would be necessary just to keep track of the requests for money. Gates kept a count for one month of all the petitions reaching his office following the announcement of a Rockefeller gift. In the first week alone, there were over fifteen thousand; by the end of the thirty days, more than fifty thousand. Rockefeller had meant what he said; all petitions were forwarded to Gates without prior screening. As Gates remembered it: "All comers, near or remote, friend or guest, high or low, were blandly sent by his ushers to my office."[18] From the first, he insisted that he remain independent of Rockefeller in all matters short of those requiring the most important decisions. Rockefeller was only too happy to comply. Gates's position within the Rockefeller establishment, then, was unique from the beginning. Although he was officially an adviser, his duties were such that he enjoyed virtual autonomy in the formulation of policy.

Although he was not yet thirty-eight when he entered Rockefeller's employ, Gates possessed a variety of experience that could be brought to bear on practically any problem within the compass of his new job. The son of a rural Baptist minister, he was born on July 2, 1853, in Maine, New York. If Stiles's self-described boyhood suggests the sunnier chapters of *Tom Sawyer,* Gates, in his seventies when he wrote his autobiography, cast his early years in a bleak, wintry light reminiscent of *Ethan Frome.* Murder, insanity, suicide, deformity, and monomaniacal religion stalked the streets of the little hamlets in which his memory placed him. His only brother, Frank, suffered from a series of illnesses throughout his childhood, the most serious of which—rheumatic fever—damaged his heart and eventually killed him. Gates tersely noted that none of the country doctors knew what to do with him. Young Gates drew back in fear and disgust from the chillingly austere religion of his father. "The orthodoxy of Calvin and Knox runs athwart our best and noblest impulses, and tends to suppress the natural instinct of right-minded persons to be friends with God," he later wrote. "The best thing that religion had to offer me as a boy was death and heaven, both of which were the very things I most dreaded, being a normal healthy boy ... All my later life I have been trying to outlive and erase my early religious training."[19] He "shrank from the publicity" of total immersion baptisms in full view of the congregation and squirmed in discomfort during the enthusiastic outbursts that punctuated his father's services. But like Stiles, as long as he was at home he was unable to slip out of the iron grip of the old-time religion and find his own intellectual footing. One tentative gesture in that direction, when he and several friends decided as a prank to try out the "anxious seat" at a Methodist revival, left him feeling "humiliated and ashamed."[20]

In the first dozen years of his life his family moved several times within the fifty-mile radius of his birthplace, but Gates remembered none of the little towns fondly. One village, Ovid, stood out in his memory only because of the rich irony he later found in its name. His father finally accepted a position with the American Home Mission Society and took his family west, first to western Missouri and soon thereafter to Kansas. Highland, Kansas, had been settled less than a decade earlier by militant New Englanders toting Beecher's Bibles. Since the end of the war, Kansas had officially stopped "bleeding," but its wounds were still too fresh to have disappeared beneath a layer of scar tissue. At Highland University, a small private school whose name expressed more accurately the dreams of its founders – a recent Dartmouth graduate and his wife – than its own modest reality, the fourteen-year-old Gates carried the day in an oratory and debating contest with a rival literary society composed exclusively of pro-Southern Missourians. The subject on the table was Women's Suffrage, and Gates argued the negative using a book by Horace Bushnell to prepare his brief.[21]

The salary of a Baptist missionary was barely adequate to support a family, much less meet tuition payments. The Gates family found itself in debt and in need of another source of income. Fred Gates left Highland University at the age of fifteen to become a schoolteacher. Not long after he left home to begin teaching, he experienced a religious conversion on his own; a pronounced continuity in his attitude toward spiritual affairs belies the notion that it was a very intense emotional one. For three years he lived frugally apart from his family, sending most of his salary home to augment his father's income. At the age of eighteen, he returned to Highland and took a position as a clerk in a dry-goods store. An uncle back east in New York had developed the "Thomas slanting steel-toothed smoothing harrow" which Gates now sold on commission to the farmers in eastern Kansas. Successful as a salesman of farm equipment, he was able to put away enough money to bring the possibility of college within reach. In the summer of 1873, when he was twenty, Gates taught himself Greek, and in September of the same year he left Highland for the relatively new university in Rochester, New York. He only stayed in Rochester for a few weeks, long enough to place completely above the freshman and sophomore years on his entrance examination. But rather than remain in Rochester to begin his junior year, Gates elected to return to Kansas for two more years of work. A Harvard graduate who ran a bank in Highland hired him to undertake, among other things, the dangerous assignment of receiving large cash deliveries at the railway station several miles away and returning, armed but alone, in a buggy to the bank—this at a time when the James and Younger gangs were operating with impunity just across the river in Missouri.[22]

In 1875 Gates made the journey east again to enroll as a junior at the University of Rochester. He soon came under the influence of Martin B. Anderson, Rochester's first president, whose tenure lasted until 1888. A New Englander whose hopes of entering the Baptist ministry were thwarted by a temporary disease of the vocal cords which prevented his speaking in public for several years, Anderson opted for teaching instead.[23] He taught rhetoric and modern history at his alma mater, Waterville College (later Colby), where he also developed a strong interest in the natural history of man. After several years of teaching, he purchased the *New York Record* and moved to Manhattan to become its editor. For over three years, he led an editorial campaign, against the opposition of many local clergymen, for the adoption of the new English translation of the Bible, but in 1853 he abruptly sold the newspaper to accept an offer of the presidency of the brand new University of Rochester. Although he stipulated when he took the job that he wished to be left free of the school's financial affairs, he soon found himself, of necessity, caught up in fundraising. He did well at it. By the time he retired thirty-five years later, Rochester's endowment and properties were worth well over a million dollars. Anderson also gained a reputation as an innovator in college curricula. He introduced and sometimes personally taught courses in psychology, art, slavery, transportation, and the relation of ethics to jurisprudence. Rochester soon became known as the place to go for a practical education in the issues of the day. Other colleges—among them Brown University, Union College, the University of Cincinnati, and the University of Michigan—offered him their presidencies, and both political parties asked him at one time or another to run for Congress, but Anderson turned aside these offers to remain at his post in Rochester.[24]

By all accounts, Anderson was a spellbinding lecturer. Gates later called his addresses "the most powerful of the formative forces on my life,"[25] and most of the evidence, at least as Gates presented it in his autobiography, bears him out. He devoted an entire chapter in his memoirs to Anderson's talks, using notes taken from letters written at the time to his parents. Anderson's philsophy was tough and practical, owing more, perhaps, to his experience as a God-fearing newspaper editor than to his days as an academic. He stressed hard work, Christian stewardship, self-reliance, discipline, humility in the face of the unknown, but above all, service to mankind. Suspicious of all theology, he held up to his students instead the goal of a life given over to practical Christianity, based on an epistemology that eschewed revelation or logic and relied on common sense for its support. One of Anderson's addresses that Gates copied out prefigures his own attitude a few years later.

We are in the midst of the unknown. We have a little bit of space about us and all the rest is darkness and mystery . . . It is true of religion, but it is true of science . . . No man is large enough, no man is learned enough to grasp all the truth in any single department of knowledge . . . Truth and error lie side by side and are involved and interlaced in countless ways. One great trouble with Theologians is they know too much. They know more than God has revealed. What neither scripture nor human consciousness give they supply by logic. When they see two truths inclining to each other like two lines nearly parallel, running a little toward each other into the darkness, they follow them into the unknown by their system of logic until they touch. And thus they fill out their systems of Theology beyond anything revealed. I am not much of a Theologian. The fact is I know less about the Bible than I did thirty years ago . . . When I see a man who has a complete system of Theology, from foundation to pinnacle, I assume at once that he is a superficial thinker . . . In my system of Theology, such that it is, the pinnacle goes way up out of sight, into the clouds of the unknown, and its foundation lies far below any vision of mine. If I could measure my system, it would not be God's.[26]

Despite Anderson's warnings and despite his own self-confessed fascination with the law, Gates chose, for reasons he never made clear, to study theology full time after his graduation from the University of Rochester. He began preparation for the Baptist ministry at the Rochester Theological School, even though he admitted that he was not "called" to the cloth. "My decision was wholly my own, and was deliberately and con-sciously reasoned." The divine voice was his own judgment. In language that sounds remarkably like Rockefeller's advice to the young man starting out in business, Gates argued: "Ideally, every man's vocation, secular or sacred alike, should be chosen in answer to the question Where can I be most useful? That, and that only is God's call to every man."[27] Anderson's strictures had planted the seeds of doubt in his mind, however, even though they did not keep him out of the seminary. He later came to view his formal religious training as a waste of time — antiquated, overly theoretical, and of no preparatory value to a pastoral ministry. His Hebrew studies, which he enjoyed, began to pose nagging questions, ignored by his instructors, concerning "the inspiration, the historic truth, and the morality of the Old Testament teaching."[28] Gates knew that a Baptist without implicit faith in the literal veracity of the Bible was not much of a Baptist at all. Still, he stuck it out for three years and in 1880, at the age of twenty-seven, entered the ministry. Shortly afterward, he was on his way west once again, to the Fifth Avenue Baptist Church of Minneapolis.

In his ordination sermon he left open the possibility of a "higher divine call." Were it to come, he told his congregation, it would "take me out of the ministry."[29] In the meantime, there were practical things to be done in Minneapolis. Of the two Baptist churches in his part of town, the Fifth Avenue was definitely the one on the wrong side of the tracks. Gates went right to work on a drive to increase the church membership with the right sort of people and to raise money for a new building. By his own estimate, and by everyone else's, his ministry was a success. Like the businessmen in his congregation, Gates tended to measure his own progress in terms borrowed from the balance sheet: the number of people baptized and enlisted on the parish rolls, the amount of money subscribed to the building fund. Even had the new church gone up on Fifth Avenue, so changed had the image of his congregation become during his pastorate that a new name would have had to be found, if only to symbolize its rebirth. As it happened, the new building was not on Fifth Avenue; located in a better part of town the parish renamed itself the Central Baptist Church.[30]

Established in Minneapolis with a thriving ministry, Gates returned to Rochester briefly in 1882 to marry Lucia Fowler Perkins. Their earlier courtship, during Gates's student days, may help to explain his decision to stay in Rochester to study for the ministry after the completion of his undergraduate work. By 1882, two years into his first call, both his position and his prospects were good enough to justify marriage. He proudly brought his bride back to the new parsonage in Minneapolis, but sixteen months later she was dead, the victim of a massive internal hemorrhage. Though Gates did not hold their family doctor directly responsible for her death, he firmly believed that the attack was not diagnosed promptly enough, or even properly. Recourse to theology offered little consolation. In fact, shortly after his wife's death, Gates abandoned it completely. "I defiantly threw overboard nearly the whole cargo that I had taken on board at the seminary, and sought to fill my little boat with the more valuable merchandise I was beginning to find . . . in the experiences of my congregation and in the study of the intellectual, spiritual, and social forces in which I lived."[31]

He began to take an active interest in the Minnesota state missions, and as he became more and more involved in their operation he came more frequently into contact with the small group of laymen, all successful Minneapolis and St. Paul businessmen, who were charged with their management. Later Gates was to remember these new associates fondly and to number them among his closest friends. The most prominent of them—indeed, the most prominent businessmen in Minnesota—came to Gates for assistance in devising a plan for a Baptist academy in the state. George A. Pillsbury, the flour manufacturer, was dying and intended to leave $200,000 in his will for the project. But he first wanted to know if there was enough interest in Minnesota to support a Baptist academy and also how the money would be used. Gates suggested, as a practical test of the public's interest, that Pillsbury announce a $50,000 gift conditioned on the willingness of Minnesota Baptists to match it. Half the money would go into the construction of buildings; the other half, into the endowment. When the school was running smoothly, Pillsbury could leave the other $150,000 in his will. Gates, who agreed to assume the responsibility for canvassing the state, was so excited by the possibilities of his new assignment that he resigned from the Central Baptist Church in March 1888 to devote all his time to fund-raising. He pursued his campaign from the pulpit and in the press, and successfully enlisted the cooperation of influential businessmen across the state. Within six weeks he had raised $60,000.[32]

A satisfied Pillsbury asked Gates to become the new school's principal. At the same time, the University of Rochester asked him to replace the retiring Anderson as its president. Gates declined both offers on the grounds that he could not imagine himself as a teacher. He accepted instead an offer to become the Executive Secretary of the new National Baptist Education Society. Recently remarried to Emma Cahoon of Racine, Wisconsin, Gates (who gained sixty pounds after he left the Central Baptist Church) prospered in his new life. Although his job was still fund-raising, his jurisdiction now included the whole country. A survey conducted under his direction of the denominational schools and colleges across the country persuaded him of the need for a large Baptist university in the Midwest, preferably on the site of the old University of Chicago, now defunct.

It was while canvassing for funds to build the new University of Chicago that Gates first approached the wealthiest Baptist of them all. Although Gates only asked for a contribution to the building fund, Rockefeller gave $100,000 in February 1889, not toward construction of the new university, but for the general educational work of the National Baptist Education Society. Four months later he did pledge $600,000 to the Chicago project, but only on condition that Gates raise another $400,000. "The raising of that four hundred thousand dollars was the most disagreeable, depressing and anxious work of my life,"[33] Gates recalled. Fourteen months earlier he had felt challenged by the task of raising $50,000; now he was charged with procuring eight times that amount. Marshall Field ensured the success of Gates' fund drive when he donated the first ten acres of the new university's property, thus publicly identifying his name with the cause. Gates crowned his success by coaxing William R. Harper, professor of Hebrew at Yale, to accept the position of president. His assignment completed, Gates himself was appointed to the Board of Trustees. A year later, Rockefeller secured the school's financial future with a gift of another $1,000,000.[34]

Although he did not yet know it, Gates had already made a strongly favorable impression on Rockefeller. Another year would pass, however, before he was summoned to New York and offered the job of principal adviser on philanthropies. Perhaps it was not good fortune as much as business necessity that kept Rockefeller alive for almost a century: he never did anything precipitately. In fact, the one year it took him to make up his mind about hiring Gates was for him a rather brief period of time to give over to an important decision. In any event, Gates unwittingly prepared himself further in that year for his future work by traveling back and forth across the country to inspect schools, confer with educators, and learn firsthand the problems they confronted. In 1891, the Lord chose John D. Rockefeller to relay "the higher divine call" Gates had foreseen in his ordination sermon eleven years earlier.

When he went to work for Rockefeller, Gates did not yet realize that he was formally renouncing his first profession, but, as he later noted, "it proved in the end that in turning my face east I was turning my back forever on the ministry."[35] The ministry was not the only aspect of his early religious life left behind in Minneapolis. He had severed his last slim tie to Baptist orthodoxy when he resigned from the Central Baptist Church. Caught up in the whirlwind of denominational fund-raising, he did not take notice of the drift his intellectual interests were following. The only book he read during this interim period in his life that left a lasting impression was Matthew Arnold's *Literature and Dogma*. Arnold re-emphasized what Gates had first heard from Anderson. "I came fully to accept the methods and the results of modern Biblical criticism and also the spirit and the results of modern scientific research. But I continued to believe that the love and good-will exemplified in the spirit of Jesus are the secret of human well-being, and that in this spirit lies the hope of the race."[36] Before he entered Rockefeller's employ, then, Gates had already come to dismiss the literal interpretation of the New Testament. When he found the Baptist minister in his new home town of Montclair, New Jersey, unacceptable by his newly developing standards, Gates and his family joined the local Congregational church.

Gates found Rockefeller's charities in a state of disarray. Most of the gifts went to Baptist churches, organizations, and missionary work, such as the National Baptist Education Society — a field he already knew well. Notwithstanding the religious character of most of the beneficiaries, Gates discovered "not a few of Mr. Rockefeller's habitual charities to be worthless and practically fraudulent." He began to apply Rockefeller's own standards more rigorously, especially since they conformed so closely to the ones he had worked out with Pillsbury and at the National Baptist Education Society. Gates preferred the term "wholesale philanthropy" to the more commonly heard "scientific giving," an indication more of his business orientation than of anything else since for all practical purposes the two terms were interchangeable. Wholesale, as opposed to retail, philanthropy eschewed outright gifts to individual units but funneled the donations through larger umbrella organizations, in much the same way that Josephine Shaw Lowell's Charity Organization Society of New York tried to prevent duplication of effort and weed out unworthy recipients. Gates would simply refer the individual petitioner back to the appropriate parent agency.[37]

Rockefeller's personal investments, randomly acquired over the years on the advice of his Baptist associates and old Cleveland friends, were in a similar state of neglect when Gates went to work for him. By 1891, there were 67 of these investments valued at $23 million. Since Gates would already be on the road a good bit of the time inspecting the widespread charities, Rockefeller asked him to undertake a "layman's" analysis of those collateral holdings which lay along his route. Gates later reviewed his qualifications for this new aspect of his job:

I was better prepared for business than Mr. Rockefeller knew, or I realized at the time. Most of my life had in fact been an unconscious preparation for successful business. My interesting experience in selling harrows, my months as a clerk in a country store, and as cashier of a country bank, my interest in my father's financial affairs and the ways and means of paying our debts, my studies of political economy under Dr. Anderson, my close study of the finances of our church building in Minneapolis, a habit of looking at things in their financial relations and tendencies as well as in other relations, my study of denominational finances at home and abroad, all these things had given me business experience and my mind a business turn.[38]

A considerable part of Rockefeller's success stemmed from his ability to choose the right associates for the particular task at hand. In Gates he had seen much more than a gregarious clergyman with a knack for balancing the parish books. He may not have known the extent of Gates's preparation when he asked him to look into his personal investments, but he had detected the streak of shrewd pragmatism behind the allegiance to high ideals. Years later, Gates was to discover in Rockefeller's personal files an old copy of a speech Gates had given in Chicago during the fund drive for the university. Rockefeller had not been among the group of Chicago businessmen in Gates's audience, but having requested a copy of the speech he saved it because of its skillful balance of pulpit-thumping Baptist oratory and cold financial analysis. In fact, oftentimes the only thing distinguishing Gates's cunning from that of Rockefeller's Standard Oil cronies was the purpose to which it was put. His rules for raising money, for example, bear this out. Drawn up in 1891 while Gates was still with the National Baptist Education Society, they illustrate the guile he could exercise, if need be, in the performance of his godly duties. Rule No. 6 cautioned would-be collectors: "If you find him [the potential donor] big with gift, do not rush too eagerly to the birth. Let him feel that he is giving it, not that it is being taken from him with violence." And Rule No. 8 advised: "Appeal only to the nobler motives. His own mind will suggest to him the lower and selfish ones. But he will not wish you to suppose that he has thought of them." Archbold could not have summoned more skill or tact in buying off a Congressman.[39]

At the time Rockefeller sought Gates's advice, he had almost written off his personal investments. He only hoped that Gates would make it easier for him to divest himself of most of them and consolidate the few he might wish to retain. Once again, just as Gates had found several of Rockefeller's charities to be spurious, he now uncovered several unsound investments. A company in Colorado set up to mine gold—a tip from a friend in Cleveland—proved, after a little judicious snooping on Gates's part, to be entirely bogus. In another case, only Rockefeller's money propped up two iron ore concerns in Alabama and Wisconsin. Rockefeller, who later called Gates's summaries "a model of what a report should be,"[40] was so pleased with the immmediate results of this detective work that he asked Gates to move into the office adjacent to his own at 26 Broadway and to pursue this new line of investigation just as assiduously as he managed the charities. Gates's general advice, which Rockefeller followed, was either to cut his losses if it appeared that a company would fail without his support or else to purchase a controlling interest if the company's prospects were favorable. Rockefeller not only gave Gates a free hand to follow his instincts but also charged him with the fortunes of the businesses acquired under the terms of the plan. In this manner Gates quickly became the president of thirteen Rockefeller-controlled corporations outside of the oil business, among them railroad lines in several different parts of the country, timber, mining, and manufacturing concerns. Gates enjoyed the traveling that had become such an integral part of his job, but he could no longer say whether the main purpose of each trip was business or philanthropy. One of his favorite interests was a mining company in the Puget Sound area, not because of its quarterly earnings but because each time he visited it he got to ride up into the Cascades on the cowcatcher of the train and to dine on brook trout which he usually caught himself.[41]

Unquestionably, Gates's most successful piece of advice was to move in and take over the Mesabi ore-producing region of northern Minnesota, where heretofore Rockefeller had only a minor interest, and to organize under his control all ore shipping on the Great Lakes. With Gates's encouragement, Rockefeller poured over $30 million into the scheme, and he hired one of Gates's uncles, L. M. Bowers—later to achieve a certain notoriety as the president of the Colorado Fuel and Iron Company at the time of the Ludlow Massacre—to oversee the construction of the ore-carrying vessels. Through a skillful series of maneuvers, Gates transformed what had been only an incidental investment into a major economic force. In a very few years, Rockefeller came to control the richest ore deposits in the world and to stand between the steel manufacturers and their raw materials at two critical points. In 1901, J. Pierpont Morgan, in the process of rationalizing the steel business, bought out the Lake Superior Consolidated Iron Mine (Frederick T. Gates, president) and its fleet of ships for $88.5 million—for the ships, $8.5 million, and for the Mesabi holdings, $80 million, half in common stock and half in preferred stock in the new United States Steel Corporation. On what had been only a passing investment of $400,000 eight years earlier, Rockefeller had made a profit of $55 million, and that before the value of the stocks began to rise.[42]

Gates's astounding business successes no doubt bolstered Rockefeller's confidence in his new philanthropic adviser. But they also ironically highlighted for Gates his major problem now that he was in the fund-dispensing and not the fund-raising business. By exercising a reasonable amount of common sense in the application of Rockefeller's huge capital as leverage, he could produce percentage returns far out of proportion to the size of the investment. But even if the holdings in Standard Oil were left to lie fallow, they still earned money at a breath-taking rate. "I was confronted with Mr. Rockefeller's fortune. He continued . . . in the habitual feelings of earlier life. He did not seem to realize . . . the immensity of his fortune. He was a born money-maker and a born money-saver. But even had it not been so, even if he had become alarmed at his colossal and every year more colossal accumulation, it was no longer in his power, from the time I first knew him, to prevent or hinder the incoming flow."[43] Between 1885 and 1896, Rockefeller's earnings from Standard Oil dividends totaled $40 million. In 1897, when he retired from the company he had founded, his net worth was estimated at $200 million. But while he was playing golf and planting trees on his Tarrytown estate, the introduction of the internal combustion engine increased the size of his fortune fivefold in fifteen years, so that by 1913, when the Standard was formally liquidated, Rockefeller was worth close to $1 billion. Carnegie had warned that "it were better for mankind that the millions of the rich were thrown into the sea" than given away impulsively. Gates found to his chagrin, however, that Rockefeller's money could make more money over a given period of time than he could disburse intelligently. They would stay in the wholesale philanthropy business, but they would have to eliminate the middlemen and set up their own spending organizations.

In the process of pruning and restructuring Rockefeller's charities and personal investments, Gates formed a friendship of sorts with his employer. To his parents he wrote that Rockefeller was "shrewd and keen and knows which end of a bargain to take hold of. He does not mean to be cheated, though he sometimes is, in the multiplicity of his business interests."[44] These were strange words of praise coming from someone who only a short time before had been holding up the Sermon on the Mount as the guide to human conduct, but from Gates they were indeed words of praise. Rockefeller himself dispensed words of praise sparingly. Gates continued to his parents: "I hear of goods words about me to others. He is confiding great interests in me, and I am exercising great caution, taking no steps until I know where my foot is going down, and whither it leads."[45] Rockefeller may not have praised Gates to his face, but he did let his opinion of his employee be known on more than one occasion, and as one might expect, it was high indeed. In his rambling autobiography, *Random Reminiscences,* serialized in *World's Work* in 1907, Rockefeller lauded Gates for "possessing a combination of rare business ability, very highly developed and very honorably exercised, overshadowed by a passion to accomplish some great and far-reaching benefits to mankind, the influence of which will last."[46] And in an interview given to B. C. Forbes, owner and editor of *Forbes Magazine,* Rockefeller cautioned: "Don't forget to explain that Mr. Gates has been the guiding genius in all our giving. He came to us first to undertake certain business matters requiring talent of a high order and he showed phenomenal business ability. He combined with this the rare quality – born, no doubt, because he had the right kind of heart – of being able to direct the distribution of money with great wisdom. We all owe much to Mr. Gates, and his helpfullness should be generously recognized. He combines business skill and philanthropic aptitude to a higher degree than any other man I have ever known."[47] Gates saved the *Forbes* article in his scrapbook of clippings after first marking in pen the passages of praise from his employer.

Gates never seems to have doubted the purity of Rockefeller's philanthropic motives. "His aim was service – service all the time, the highest service, and that disinterested."[48] Perhaps the service itself was disinterested, but Gates had solid evidence that Rockefeller was not unmoved by the consequences of his gifts. Gates recalled in a letter to Charles W. Eliot, "I have seen the tears of joy course down his cheeks as he contemplated the past achievement and future possibilities" of his philanthropies.[49]

Very few other people saw Rockefeller express emotion of any kind. In fact, to those who knew them both, Gates was the emotional one, and Rockefeller his exact opposite. Raymond Fosdick described the contrast:

One would have to search over wide areas to find two men who were so completely different in temperament. Mr. Gates was a vivid, outspoken, self-revealing personality who brought an immense gusto to his work; Mr. Rockefeller was quiet, cool, taciturn about his thoughts and purposes, almost stoic in his repression. Mr. Gates had an eloquence which could be passionate when he was aroused; Mr. Rockefeller, when he spoke at all, spoke in a slow measured fashion, lucidly and penetratingly, but without raising his voice and without gestures. Mr. Gates was overwhelming and sometimes overbearing in argument; Mr. Rockefeller was a man of infinite patience who never showed irritation or spoke chidingly about anybody. Mr. Gates summed up his impression of Mr. Rockefeller in this sentence: "If he was very nice and precise in his choice words, he was also nice and accurate in his choice of silences."[50]

Beneath their differences, however, the two men had much in common. Both had been born in rural upstate New York before the Civil War into evangelical Baptist families; both had moved west with their families at about the same age; both started working for a living in their mid-teens; and both returned to New York in middle life after successful starts in the Midwest.

In 1897, another man destined to play a major role in the development and management of the extensive philanthropic network joined the Rockefeller organization. John D. Rockefeller, Jr. graduated from Brown University in that year and, at the age of twenty-three, elected to forgo law school and a trip around the world in order to begin working in his father's business as soon as possible. "I felt that I had no time for either," he wrote; "that if I was going to learn to help Father in the care of his affairs, the sooner my apprenticeship under his guidance began, the better."[51] In point of fact, young Rockefeller served most of his apprenticeship under Gates. Never as tough as his father and without the serene moral self-confidence, the thick skin, and the love of competition that enabled the elder Rockefeller to thrive in the business world for seven decades, Rockefeller, Jr. had to endure several painful and humiliating public experiences between 1900 and 1915 before finally deciding that his future lay exclusively in the management of the philanthropies. By that time, most of the important decisions defining the goals of the Rockefeller charities for the next half-century, and creating the means for their achievement, had already been made.

The loose, three-cornered partnership between the two Rockefellers and Gates functioned for twenty years as the nucleus of the multifarious activities supported by Rockefeller funds. The older Rockefeller was never actively involved in the operation of the philanthropies set up after his retirement, but he maintained a lively interest in the general direction of the benefactions made in his name and retained, in theory at least, the right of final approval. Rockefeller, Jr., although he did not emerge as the man in charge until after the goals had been set and the working principles institutionalized, did shoulder a large share of the administrative duties for the programs initiated after the turn of the century. He was also personally responsible for setting in motion the sequence of events that led to the formation of the General Education Board. But if the organizations set up after 1900 bear the stamp of any one man, that man is Gates. Not only did he direct the day-to-day affairs of the principal philanthropies, at least until the creation of the Rockefeller Foundation in 1913, but he also, more than either of his partners, chose the types of projects to be supported by Rockefeller donations. A glance at the difference between Rockefeller's denominational charities from the days before Gates's arrival and the medical and educational programs of the early 1900s will give a good indication of the extent to which Gates was much more than just the brilliant but passive instrument of the Rockefellers' will. Rockefeller, Jr., a self-effacing man even after he came into his own, was being accurate, and not modest, when he later said: "Gates was the brilliant dreamer and creator. I was the salesman."[52]

# 4

# Philanthropy for
# the Ages

The Rockefeller Sanitary Commission for the Eradication of Hookworm Disease was a direct, lineal descendant of two early organizations developed under the careful cultivation of Gates and Rockefeller, Jr. Each helped to shape different aspects of the Commission's approach to the problem of hookworm in the South. The Rockefeller Institute for Medical Research (founded in 1901) provided a basis of interest in scientific medicine and public health, while the General Education Board (charted in 1903) furnished an elite corps of Southerners experienced in dealing with the needs of the "forgotten man" in their native region. The General Education Board also gave Gates and Rockefeller, Jr. a practical introduction to the intricacies of running a philanthropic enterprise in the Southern states.

Gates developed an interest in the possibility of creating an institution devoted entirely to medical research after reading William Osler's *Principles and Practice of Medicine.* A young medical student in New York, who as a child had been a parishioner of Gates's in Minneaspolis, gave him a copy to read in July 1897. Gates was already predisposed to view the medical profession in the United States with skepticism. He had lost both a brother and a wife at young ages, and, in his opinion, neither attending physician had been of much value. His mistrust of doctors grew during his days in Minneapolis and kept pace with his theological doubts. Before he left the clergy, he had come to believe that "if there existed a science of medicine, that science was not being taught in the United States." Osler intrigued him. "I read the whole book without skipping any of it . . . There was a fascination about the style that led me on, and having once started, I found a hook in my nose that pulled me from page to page." Osler's style was not the only aspect of the book that captured and held his attention. Gates found his own skepticism borne out in Osler's conclusions. There were hundreds of diseases recognized by the mid-1890s, Osler contended, but the average physician with a normal practice could count on his fingers the number he could actually cure. "I came at length to approach his [Osler's] curative suggestions with a smile . . . He would suggest that such and such celebrated physicians . . . found this or that treatment was efficacious, but such had not been his own experience."[1]

Gates came away from his cram course in the problems of contemporary medicine with an even gloomier opinion of its extent and precision, especially in the United States. The elder Rockefeller agreed that American medicine needed a stimulus toward modernization. Like Gates, he too had lost members of his immediate family at early ages—in his case, a younger sister and a daughter. In 1901, scarlet fever carried off his first grandchild. Despite his personal, life-long loyalty to an unreconstructed homeopath—a constant source of irritation to Gates, who was convinced tha Dr. H. F. Biggar whispered heresies in his patient's ear—Rockefeller was easily persuaded to endow an institute for scientific research in medicine along the lines of the Koch Institute in Berlin and the Pasteur Institute in Paris. He and Gates both believed that if such a haven for pure medical research could be set up in America, it might serve as a catalyst for the stimulation and development of a modern approach to medicine in all parts of the country.[2]

Rockefeller certainly had the resources to underwrite an institute conceived on such a grand scale, but no amount of money could create overnight an American medical scientist of Robert Koch's or Louis Pasteur's stature around whom such an enterprise could be organized. That person simply did not exist in the United States at the turn of the century. What America did have in comparative abundance, however, were men who excelled in the mobilization of other people's energies and ideas. The special contributions that Americans made toward the modernization of science and technology early in the twentieth century lay more in the application, the engineering, the institutionalization of new knowledge. Thus the United States produced a Henry Ford, not a Carl Friedrich Benz; a G. Stanley Hall, not a Sigmund Freud; a Thomas Alva Edison, not a James Clerk Maxwell; a Robert Millikan, not an Albert Einstein. In the absence of an American Koch or Pasteur, Gates found William Henry Welch and Simon Flexner.

William Henry Welch, fifty-one years old when he took up his duties as president of the Rockefeller Institute, was already the pre-eminent figure in American medicine. Within his lifetime Welch witnessed, and to a great extent guided, the transformation of medicine in the United States from a woefully imprecise, unspecialized pseudoscience into today's network of vast hospital and teaching complexes, using highly trained and highly differentiated specialists, and placing greatly increased emphasis on technology and research. Welch's importance within the medical profession was not based on original ideas or discoveries, but rather on his abilities as a teacher, organizer, leader, and promoter of scientific medicine. Most of his career centered on the Johns Hopkins medical school. After several years as an instructor of pathology at Bellevue Hospital Medical College, he went to Baltimore in 1884 as one of the first professors on the Johns Hopkins faculty, and in 1893 he became the first dean of the new medical school. More than any of the other founders, Welch was responsible for assembling the great faculty in medicine at John Hopkins and for designing its curriculum.[3]

Simon Flexner, the first director of the Rockefeller Institute, had taken an M.D. degree from the University of Louisville in 1889 and a year later, at his brother Abraham's suggestion, entered Johns Hopkins for postgraduate work in pathology and bacteriology under Welch. When the Johns Hopkins medical school opened it doors two years later, Welch asked Flexner to be his first assistant in the department of pathology. He left the job for more study abroad in Strasbourg and Prague, and later took a position at the University of Pennsylvania medical school, where he organized and recruited the staff and planned the new laboratory building. Although he thought of himself primarily as a pathologist, Flexner's real strength was as an administrator. He was one of the first men in the United States to understand and put into effect the idea of team research, with its integrated system of specialized departments and laboratories. Under this type of working arrangement, a bacteriologist, for example, is kept abreast of the work of a biochemist in another part of the research center through regularly scheduled staff meetings, discussions, and lectures. Unlike its European precursors, the Rockefeller Institute, under Flexner's guidance, did not stake out one particular area of medicine as its field of endeavor, but rather brought together under one roof researchers in several different medical subdivisions, organized into separate departments, each under the direction of a scientist *qua* administrator. Flexner encouraged each member of his staff to pursue his special field of interest, but at the same time he tried to keep the barriers between departments as low as possible. Gates wrote of is contribution to the success of the Institute: "Dr. Flexner has every quality, without exception, of the masterful executive, while retaining the devotion and loyalty of his associates and subordinates. It is nothing but simple truth to say that the Rockefeller Institute has not been less fortunate in its great administrator than in its great founder."[4]

Gates's comparison may not be quite as farfetched as it appears at first glance. Rockefeller had employed very similar organizational and entrepreneurial skills in the process of monopolizing the oil industry. "Oil," in Daniel Boorstin's words, "offered fantastic new opportunities, and the man who organized these opportunities was a Go-Getter of heroic proportions."[5] Flexner's administrative talents were likewise employed in organizing the research opportunities open to the scientists he brought to work at the Institute. Some members of the staff, most notably Paul de Kruif, found Flexner overbearing and difficult to work with, but Alexis Carrel, the Institute's first Nobel laureate, expressed the sentiments of most of his colleagues when he wrote to Flexner: "The Rockefeller Institute is yourself. You are its mind."[6]

If Carrel had located the Institute's mind, Gates was sure he had glimpsed its soul. Usually the model of cool restraint when it came to the actual disbursement of funds and the implementation of philanthropic programs, Gates had been impatient from the moment Rockefeller gave his consent to see the Institute built and under way. In 1926, as he was writing his autobiography, he looked back fondly on the Institute as the grandest achievement in all his years with the Rockefellers, eclipsing in his estimation the Foundation itself. Flexner, Welch, and the others might gauge the Institute's achievements in purely scientific terms and take a just pride in what they saw. Gates was not oblivious to this component of its success, of course, but for him, as for no one else intimately connected with its life, the Institute satisfied a distinctly religious need.

Gates had begun his slow climb of Mencken's golden spires years earlier when he was still a seminary student, and he fully believed that by keeping his eyes and his mind open he had finally exorcised the primeval rain-god of his youth. He still called himself a Christian, but his religion was "simply the service of humanity in the Spirit of Jesus." So undoctrinaire a faith did not balk at the nineteenth-century scientific discoveries. To Gates,

"Creeds, churches, sects, religious organizations, and all the agencies of civilization are to be valued and used only as they are agents in the service of humanity on earth."[7] It was not simply that he instinctively preferred the just and rational Jesus of Luke the Physician to the Jehovah of Jeremiah; he also believed that civilized men in the early twentieth century no longer needed to be bullied and threatened like wayward children into doing what was right and good. To Gates Christian ethics were all the more illuminating once they were taken out of the shadow of the Old Testament God of wrath and judgment. They ensured that human progress would proceed in the right direction. And science, steadily pushing back the boundaries of Martin Anderson's "little bit of clear space about us," guaranteed that humanity would progress through "an even closer approach to the facts, the laws, the forces of nature." Of all the sciences, medical research—most obviously in the service of mankind—was the most progressive. Far from being mutually exclusive, then, medical research and the teachings of Jesus actually complemented and reinforced each other. Charles Sheldon, author of the extremely popular *In His Steps*, had not included a medical researcher among his characters, each of whom asked himself before making a practical decision in the course of his daily affairs, "What would Jesus do?" In Gates's opinion, pieced together from his statements in the autobiography, the mere fact of the scientist's presence in the laboratory would have been enough to satisfy Jesus.

Though Gates denied God the dreadful power of caprice over his own life, he was yet orthodox enough, despite his ostensible liberation, to believe that there still existed a mysterious and majestic God out there in the darkness somewhere. If He no longer had to chasten, His will to make known, it was because mankind no longer had to rely on the frail and imprecise instrument of formal logic to interpret His wishes. The scientists at the Institute might think that their beacon only cast its light horizontally across the surface of the material world into the corners of ignorance and the crevices of disease. Gates, however, had detected another beam, originating in the same source, but pointed vertically, up into the heavens. "I hesitate to speak of another thing that makes this Institute highly interesting to me. Do not smile if I say that I often think of this Institute as a sort of Theological Seminary . . . In these sacred rooms He is whispering His secrets. To these men He is opening up the mysterious depths of His Being." The scientists at the Institute were not just the watchmen telling of the night to the rest of humankind. They were also the new elect. Gates believed that "if there be over us all the Sum of All . . . and that Being has any favorites on this little planet . . . those favorites are made up of that ever-enlarging group of men and women who are most intimately and in very truth studying Him and His ways with men."[8]

The religious significance of the work of the Institute was of an even more palpable and personal kind to Gates. As a boy in his father's church, he had been constitutionally unable to take refuge in the nonrational side of evangelical Protestantism; he had been too self-conscious and too uncomfortable to experience a sense of wonder, an exquisite trembling, in the presence of God. His later identification of what he perceived to be superstitions and errors in the theological underpinnings of his Baptist faith, and the painstaking redefinition of his religious convictions made the prospects of that kind of emotional surrender seem even more remote. But now in the laboratories of the Rockefeller Institute the scales had fallen away from his eyes, and those scales were lens caps. "There have been times when, as I have looked through these microscopes, I have been stricken with speechless awe. I have felt that I have been gazing with unhallowed eyes into the secret places of the Most High . . . even though clouds and darkness are round about Him."[9]

Gates came back down from the cloud-wreathed summit of Mount Sinai with no stone tablets, but full of hope. The moral of medical research, even to those who had not seen the face of God through a microscope, was revolutionary in its implications.

As medical research goes on . . . it will find out and promulgate, as an unforeseen by-product of its work, new moral laws and new social laws — new definitions of what is right and wrong in our relations with each other. Medical research will educate the human conscience in new directions and point out new duties. It will make us sensitive to new moral distinctions. It will teach nobler conceptions of our social relations and of the God who is over us all. Work being done in the Institute may be far more important than we dream, for the ethics and the religion of the future.[10]

But outmoded theologies based on human logic had often prescribed sound codes of human conduct. Granted, a moral law rooted in the discoveries of science would be truer to the natural order and, to an admirer of the scientific approach to the abiding mysteries of the universe, presumably more complete. Medical research, however, could accomplish, in Gates's view, what all the theologies in the world could not. It could construct that overarching system that Anderson had stopped sort of contemplating. "The work of the Institute is as universal in its scope as the love of God. It goes to the fountains of life itself. It deals with what is innermost in every man. And while we think of the universality of its scope . . . let us remember its permanency. The work is not for today alone, but forever; not for this generation, but for every generation of humanity that shall come after us. Thus every success is multiplied by infinity."[11]

The men in the laboratories overlooking the East River, one of whom was Gates's oldest son, were engaged in something far larger than they imagined, and Gates's patron had wrought far more than he knew. The profits from Standard Oil would yet redress the accumulated shortcomings of millennia and make straight in the desert a highway toward the Millennium yet to come. The twentieth century would succeed where the sixteenth century had failed, now that John Rockefeller's Institute had superseded John Calvin's *Institutes*.

Of the three spheres – science, philanthropy, and education – that coalesced to give body and direction to the Rockefeller Sanitary Commission, two were brought together in the Institute for Medical Research. At the same time this union was developing into a working reality, the Rockefeller charities were taking the preliminary steps into the province of education, with a special emphasis on education in the South. The General Education Board brought within the perimeter of the Rockefeller establishment several renowned Southern educators, acutely aware of the special needs of their region and experienced in dealing with its people. One of these special problems, as Stiles well knew but as the others did not yet realize, stemmed directly from the high incidence of hookworm infection indigenous to the South. Owing to the very nature of hookworm disease and the manner in which it spread, any systematic crusade to bring about its eradication would have to be waged with a two-edged sword. Not only would the immediate sufferers have to be cured, but the general population would also have to be indoctrinated in the ways to prevent its recurrence. Rockefeller money bridged the gap between science and education in this particular endeavor, but the existence of two organizations under the Rockefeller aegis prior to the formation of the Sanitary Commission – one working in the realm of medical research, the other in the field of education – enabled the fusion to occur even more easily.

Inadequate public education was one of the more glaring deficiencies in Southern society at the turn of the century. According to the United States census of 1900, there were 1,198,774 illiterate native whites and 2,637,774 illiterate blacks ten years of age or older. Roughly 12 percent of the Southern white population could not read or write, against a national average of 4.6 percent. Black illiteracy had dropped by a remarkable one-third in the twenty-year period ending in 1900, but it still stood at an appalling 50 percent.[12]

Since the Civil War, the lack of public schooling in the Southern states had been a source of concern for zealous Northern philanthropists, most of whom believed that widespread literacy for both races would help to forestall the reimposition of a planter-dominated hierarchical society. The slave owners themselves had indirectly furnished evidence to support the contentions of their enemies when they wrote into the slave codes prohibitions against the most rudimentary instruction. When Union guns detached the South Carolina Sea Islands from the Confederacy only seven months after the firing on Fort Sumter, a motley but determined and high-minded contingent of philanthropists, missionaries, and schoolteachers from Massachusetts and New York quickly put into effect their own ad hoc reconstruction program among the ten thousand freedmen there, long before Lincoln had formulated a coherent plan of his own — indeed, long before other Northern military successes made such a plan seem necessary.[13]

Shortly after the war, George Peabody, a Massachusetts-born London banker and philanthropist, established a fund of some $2 million for the "promotion and encouragement of intellectual, moral, or industrial education among the young of the more destitute portions of the Southern and Southwestern States of our Union . . . without other distinction than their needs and the opportunities of usefulness to them."[14] Peabody had been active for years in public housing schemes in London as well as in cultural projects in the United States, but the Civil War made the need for more museums seem, from his vantage point three thousand miles away, much less urgent. England had for years drained wealth in the form of cotton out of the South; now a shrewd American businessman would see to it that some English money found its way back across the Atlantic to the Southern states at a time when they most needed it. The legendary Southern hospitality made the prospect of a worthy enterprise on behalf of the suffering people even more pleasing for Peabody to contemplate. He had enjoyed several congenial and prosperous years in Baltimore before moving to London and had more recently returned, four years before the outbreak of hostilities, to tour the South, where he had received "the most kind and flattering attentions from every city" he visited. Over the next four-and-a-half decades, a glittering array of national figures, evenly balanced between Northerners and Southerners, graced the board of trustees of the Peabody Fund. General Grant was among the members of the original group; and as the early participants died or retired they were replaced by other, almost as prominent, Americans, including three other Presidents, two Chief Justices, and J. Pierpont Morgan, a branch of government unto himself.[15]

The other major educational fund in the South before the turn of the century came into being in 1882 following a $1 million gift to improve black education from John F. Slater, a Connecticut textile manufacturer. The Slater Fund's roster of trustees rivaled the Peabody's in prestige; in fact, several of the same names appeared on both. Venerable features of the Southern educational system by the time Rockefeller entered the field, the Peabody and Slater Funds had made a small dent in Southern illiteracy, as the difference in the census figures between 1880 and 1900 suggests.[16]

Rockefeller's concern for the plight of Southern blacks was as old as his involvement in philanthropy. In his youth he had been surrounded by strong abolitionist sentiment in pre-Civil War Ohio, and his wife's family had taken an active part in the work of the underground railroad. One of the earliest entries in his Ledger A recorded a donation to help a free black in Cleveland buy his wife out of slavery. Although the Baptist educational societies he later supported devoted most of their attention to white denominational schools in the South and the Midwest, Rockefeller himself had had directly underwritten a Baptist seminary for black girls in Atlanta, later renamed Spelman College in honor of his wife's family. He had encouraged his children when they were young to visit Hampton Institute, a black college in Virginia, where each had "adopted" a needy student. In 1901, then, he was not averse to his son's acceptance of an invitation to attend the fourth Conference on Southern Education, to be held that year in Winston-Salem, North Carolina.[17]

Rockefeller, Jr. journeyed to the conference aboard a train chartered for the occasion by the chairman, Robert Curtis Ogden. An associate of John Wanamaker and the manager of his New York store, Ogden had also helped to found Hampton Institute. At the time of the Winston-Salem meeting, he was the president of its board of trustees and a member of the Tuskegee Institute's governing board as well. Ogden was the very image of Ralph Ellison's aged Yankee philanthropist in the early chapters of *Invisible Man.* His chartered trains, of which the one in 1901 was the first, formed the reconnaissance and promotional arm of what came to be known as the "Ogden movement." Although it made stops all over the South—at Hampton Institute, Atlanta University, the Tuskegee Institute, all black schools financed with Northern money—the "millionaires' special," as Ogden's train was called in Southern newspapers, picked up most of its passengers in New York. The younger Rockefeller's traveling companions numbered over forty and included Walter Hines Page (editor of *World's Work* magazine), George Foster Peabody (a Georgia-born New York banker, not to be confused with the George Peabody of the Peabody Fund), Albert Shaw (editor of *Review of Reviews*), William H. Baldwin, Jr. (president of the Long Island Railroad), and Lyman Abbott (editor of *The Outlook*). The special guests on Ogden's package tour stopped in Winston-Salem just long enough to meet with other delegates from across the South, who presumably had dug into their own pockets and consulted the standard timetables to reach the conference. They all endorsed a proposal to initiate "a campaign of education for free schools for all people," regardless of color, but since no one knew quite where or how to begin, the conference closed after elevating Ogden to the presidency of whatever organization he saw fit to create in order to carry out their resolution.[18]

Ogden began by forming a committee. It included J. L. M. Curry, the redoubtable former Congressman, ex-rebel, and long-time Special Agent of the Peabody Fund; Charles W. Dabney, president of the University of Tennessee; Hollis B. Frissell, principal of Hampton Institute; Edwin A. Alderman, president of Tulane University; Wallace Buttrick, chairman of the American Baptist Home Mission Society's committee on education; and George Foster Peabody. Shaw, Page, and Baldwin were later added to the list of directors of the new organization, which called itself the Southern Education Board. With only a $30,000 gift from George Foster Peabody to work with, the Board had to start by setting its sights rather low. Its sole avowed purpose, as defined by its original directors, was to lobby enthusiastically on behalf of tax-supported schools in the South. That the nature and the scope of the Southern Education Board's operations broadened considerably over the course of its fourteen-year life was no doubt due to the way in which the Rockefeller men chose to use it, a way that must have appealed to the old architect of Standard Oil—that is, as a dummy corporation.[19]

The younger Rockefeller had left Winston-Salem for the trip home inflamed with the idea of forming an organization to promote black education in the South. His plans were drastically modified before they even had a chance to become much more than pipe dreams, however, by a warning from Henry St. George Tucker, president of Washington and Lee College, who boarded the train on its way north through Virginia specifically, it seems, to disabuse its passengers of any misguided, idealistic notions they might have acquired on the trip, before they got back to New York and did something foolish. It was all well and good that they were filled with concern for the Southern blacks, Tucker told them, but "if it is your idea to educate the Negro, you must have the white of the South with you. If the poor white sees the son of a Negro neighbor enjoying through your munificence benefits denied to his boy, it raises in him a feeling that will render futile all your work."[20] Tucker was a persuasive Cassandra. He did not need to go into a detailed explanation of the possible ways in which the poor white might choose to act on the feeling thus raised. The Slater Fund had been set up twenty years earlier, a time that by 1900 seemed like a halcyon period in Southern race relations. Since then, frustrated Populists, New South boosters, and demagogues alike had fostered their various interests by exacerbating racial tensions with a fury that grew in intensity throughout the 1890s. By the beginning of the twentieth century, a legal segregation more thorough and more stringent than anything envisioned by the slave owners reached into every corner of Southern life. Frissell at Hampton and Booker T. Washington at Tuskegee had enjoyed a degree of success precisely because they recognized the Southern order of things and had accommodated their educational programs to it. Washington had publicly acknowledged the new order not five years earlier in his Atlanta speech, shortly before the United States Supreme Court sanctified it in the *Plessy* v. *Ferguson* decision. Unless the Northern philanthropists were careful in their choice of ways to promote their good intentions, they would yet make a prophet out of Mississippi's Senator James K. Vardaman, who had said: "What the North is sending the South is not money, but dynamite."[21]

Despite Tucker's stern lesson in Southern social realities, Rockefeller, Jr. still regarded the trip as "one of the outstanding events of my life." Out of his modified enthusiasm came the first steps leading to the creation of the General Education Board. On February 27, 1902, ten men met in his home to pledge their support and to sign a statement in which they contracted to use $1 million his father had promised to meet educational needs all over the country over the next ten years. Seven of the ten men had only months earlier pledged to spend George Foster Peabody's $30,000 in much the same way. Why would Gates and the elder Rockefeller, with their abhorrence of waste in all forms, including duplication of effort, consent to enter the field hard on the heels of another organization committed to the same goals? The fact that Rockefeller, Jr. had been left off Ogden's board of directors, despite his keenness to work for educational reform, indicates that plans were already afoot to set up the General Education Board, even as the Southern Education Board was coming into existence. Moreover, Ogden and Peabody, the prime movers in the formation of the Southern Education Board, were among the men gathered in Rockefeller, Jr.'s home on February 27 and were signatories to the General Education Board's statement of purpose. Had they and the others resented the appearance of a powerful and much larger rival, they would hardly have assisted at its birth.[22]

Gates and the two Rockefellers were obviously eager to enter the field of educational philanthropy in a big way, and they no doubt wanted to control whatever program they financed. But their desire for anonymity in this instance outweighed their desire for control and goes further toward an explanation of their choice of methods. The Southern Education Board, with the complicity of its founders, would be their stalking horse until the General Education Board was firmly on its own feet. Rockefeller's name might adorn a self-contained institute for medical research, the success of which was not dependent on public support, but a large effort to promote and improve public education would require the cooperation of hundreds of thousands of people not on the Rockefeller payroll, many of whom thought of Rockefeller as an archfiend. The absence of the family name on the new organization, and the pledge to work for education everywhere in the country though the directors knew they were bound by the terms of the gift to focus their early efforts on the South, made it easier for Nelson Aldrich of Rhode Island, the younger Rockefeller's father-in-law and the Republican leader of the United States Senate, to guide a bill through Congress on January 12, 1903, chartering the General Education Baord and permitting it to hold unlimited capital. Before it undertook specific programs in its own right, however, the General Education Board channeled money earmarked for promotional work in the South through the Southern Education Board in order to prepare the ground for its own harvests to come. In the next twelve years approximately $100,000 in Rockefeller funds, twice laundered in this manner, flowed into public relations efforts in the Southern states, much of it in the first few years of the General Education Board's existence. But $100,000, though a major part of the Southern Education Board's budget, was only a fraction of the General Education Board's expenditures in its first decade. Its commitments ramified so quickly and its labors proved so fruitful by its own standards that Rockefeller's initial pledge of $1 million was swallowed up in the $16 million actually appropriated and the over $30 million placed at the Board's disposal before June 30, 1914. The elephant soon gave up trying to hide in the mouse's shadow. By 1921 Rockefeller had given almost $130 million to expand and to sustain the activities of the General Education Board, the largest educational organization of its kind in the world.[23]

Since Gates selected Wallace Buttrick (1853-1926) to be the Board's first secretary, it is not surprising that Buttrick was a man like Gates in many respects. He too had been born in upstate New York in 1853 – in Potsdam, on October 23. He too had worked (as a railway mail clerk) to pay his way through the Rochester Theological Seminary, which he entered at his wife's urging and from which he graduated in 1882, two years after Gates. He too entered the parish ministry after seminary and served as pastor for churches in New Haven, St. Paul (not far from Gates's parish in Minneapolis), and Albany, before he turned to fund-raising and philanthropic administration. While a parish minister, Buttrick also served as a trustee of the University of Rochester and of the Rochester Theological Seminary. One wonders how often his parishioners actually got a chance to hear him preach, for in this same period he served on the executive board of the American Baptist Home Mission Society and was the chairman of its committe on education. For a time, he worked as a general agent for the Slater Fund. His path had crossed Gates's many times over a period of twenty years before Gates asked him to come to work for the General Education Board. Like Gates, Buttrick was first and foremost a businessman, much of whose heart, even while he was a parish minister, remained in the marketpace. A fellow clergyman once asked him for his idea of heaven. Buttrick replied without hesitation, "My office!"[24]

Buttrick saw little of his office in his first few years at the General Education Board. Though (or perhaps because) he had a million dollars at his disposal, he did not know how to begin to spend it. Casting about for a plan of operation that would satisfy the Rockefellers' principles of giving without outraging Southerners, Buttrick travelled widely through the South from 1902 to 1905. "We shall err and invite defeat," he cautioned, in words that echoed Tucker's, "if in the present state of public sentiment, we demand too much from the white people of the South."[25] The cities and towns clearly offered the best hope of immediate rewards with less risk, but 85 percent of the Southern population lived in the countryside. The early General Education Board grants—small, tentative, haphazard—reflected Buttrick's indecision. Gates was nominally a trustee from the moment of the Board's inception, but he was far too preoccupied with the plans for the Institute for Medical Research to come to Buttrick's assistance right away. By 1905, however, his scientists were hard at work in temporary quarters while their permanent home rapidly neared completion, and Gates could turn his attention to the problems of the General Education Board. Not one to wait patiently for an opening to present itself once a program was supposedly under way, Gates deplored what he called the Board's "policy of scatteration." Not surprisingly, the Board took its first large and confident steps shortly after Gates began looking for an opportunity.[26]

The General Education Board was the direct precursor of the Sanitary Commission in certain important attitudes, procedural methods, and personnel. Although the Institute came into being at the same time and provided a ready pool of medical and scientific experience, the General Education Board was without question the Commission's most important progenitor since the problem of hookworm disease was more an educational than a purely medical one. Both the Institute and the Board operated under the patronage of the Rockefeller philanthropies and both in their early stages owed much to Frederick Gates's vision, but here the fundamental similarities between the sister organizations ended. Whereas the Institute was basically an autonomous unit—answering specific needs of elements within the general population, to be sure, but answering them in the laboratory rather than in the field—the work of the General Education Board necessitated direct contact with the people involved at the locus of the problem, not in a self-contained medical complex in New York. The duties of the Board, unlike those of the Institute, required that a working rapport between benefactors and beneficiaries be established along clearly defined guidelines. Rockefeller's four tenets governing philanthropic expenditures provided the philosophical basis for these guidelines, but the peculiar nature of the undertaking, as seen by Gates and Buttrick, determined the specific form they ultimately assumed. A study of the Rockefeller Sanitary Commission should include a look at some of the General Education Board's early experiences since they foreshadowed and, to some extent, determined the goals and methods of the campaign against hookworm disease.

Although it did help to finance the construction of new primary and secondary schools, the General Education Board carried out the major portion of its work in the South through existing institutions. Early subsidies went to Southern teachers' colleges, partially because it was easier to make gifts of this kind unobtrusively, but also because the officers of the Board realized that new schoolhouses were of little value without teachers to staff them. Financially weak or irresponsible colleges receiving General Education Board funds were often required to submit their books to the Rockefeller auditors. But although it required fiscal responsibility, the Board never overtly demanded that an institution raise a certain sum of money. At the same time, it never gave the entire amount needed for a specific project, either. Gates had first suggested this formula to Pillsbury almost twenty years earlier as a good practical test of a community's commitment. He himself had been bound by the same conditions in connection with the funding of the University of Chicago. The General Education Board's allotments—ususally one-half, but sometimes one-third or one-fourth—were offered on a comparable grant-in-aid basis. The gift was not directly contingent on the institution's ability to match it—it would not be withdrawn if the rest of the needed sum were not raised—but the burden of responsibility fell on the shoulders of the beneficiary. This loose, unwritten plan worked remarkably well. No evidence has yet been found to indicate that an institution ever needed coercion to meet its obligations. The usual pattern was for the trustees of a school or the town fathers to set a specific goal for a specific purpose and only then to ask the General Education Board for a contribution.[27]

Gates and Buttrick also devised a plan to circumvent recalcitrant state legislatures and to lobby on the local level for primary and secondary schools, without showing Rockefeller's hand. Starting in 1905 at the University of Virginia where a cooperative President Alderman, fresh from Tulane, smoothed the way, the General Education Board donated the funds to pay a professor of secondary education whose chief duty was "to ascertain where . . . the conditions are favorable for the establishment of public high schools not now in existence."[28] He began by conducting a state-wide survey designed to produce a clear picture of the present state of secondary education within his jurisdiction. Only after he had completed the survey did he begin to work in individual communities, talking up the idea of a high school. No one in town need know that his salary and expenses were picked up by the Rockefellers; his credentials only read that he was on the faculty of the state university and that his specialty was secondary education. Only after he had persuaded the citizens of a community that they should raise the money to build a high school, or improve an existing one, or add a fourth year to a three-year one, or consolidate with a neighboring town, or free a high school teacher from responsibilities with the younger students, would the professor of secondary education mention that he knew of a national organization which might be willing to donate a portion of the money they needed – and then only if it appeared that the town could not raise it all without outside help. In most instances he never had to mention the General Education Board at all.

By the end of 1908, ten states had professors of secondary education, each a carefully chosen young Southerner who held a dual appointment at the university and at the state department of education. Copies of his reports went to his two offices and to the central office of the General Education Board as well. In addition, each professor of secondary education became perforce something of a lobbyist in the state capital, pushing for enabling legislation to permit towns to levy taxes to implement the ideas he had already sown. In 1905, when the first such professor was appointed, the General Education Board found that "the four-year high school, properly so-called, was practically nonexistent in the South outside a few large towns," and "that in general the high school was for the most part vague and formless."[29] By June 30, 1914, after a decade of work, it could report that although "the term 'high school' does not yet mean the same thing or the same sort of thing everywhere, it is nowadays used in the South with a fair degree of critical caution."[30] To document this change of attitudes, the General Education Board pointed to the 1,237 new high schools—625 four-year and 612 three-year—established since 1905. Its own contribution to their construction and operating budgets had been a relatively modest $242,816.09, or about 1 percent of the total amount expended. The vast bulk of the funds so used had come from a combination of legislative apportionments, private contributions, and local education taxes. Gates was so impresed with the early returns on his small investment that he quickly put into effect a parallel program, headed by a group of new officials titularly under the state superintendents of public education but in fact paid by the Board, to do the same sort of thing for primary education in rural areas.[31]

Even if the people in a rural community were eager to see their new schools succeed, unless they themselves prospered their schools stood little chance. Buttrick later admitted that, at the outset, he and the trustees had naively "thought that a schoolhouse with a teacher constituted a school, and that if we could only multiply schoolhouses and schools in sufficient numbers, the problem of education would be solved.'[32] Gates was probably the first person on the General Education Board to recognize that the sad state of Southern education was less a consequence of general apathy than a function of poverty. And since the region's economic system, despite two decades of New South propaganda, still rested squarely on agriculture, the Board would have to address itself to the problem of farm productivity if it wished to see its educational improvements maintained. The connection between rural poverty and school tax revenues became obvious once one stopped and thought about it. After a 1905 visit to Hampton Institute, someone asked Gates what he thought of a new dairy farm he had seen on the campus. Gates answered as though he had been reading John Taylor of Caroline all his life: "If that land will support that barn, it is a good thing. But if that land will not support that barn, it is a bad thing."[33] What was true of dairy barns was just as true of public schools.

While he was screening prospective professors of secondary education, Gates was also searching for "a practical way" to introduce Southern farmers to "the science and art of agriculture," something a few Southerners in each generation had been trying to do with little success since the days of the Virginia Company. Buttrick went back on the road at Gates's behest, scouring the agricultural colleges of Canada, the Midwest, and the South for over eight months before David F. Houston, president of Texas A&M, introduced him to Seaman A. Knapp. Another transplanted upstate New Yorker, Knapp was already seventy-three years old and well launched on his seventh successful career when Buttrick met him. In earlier professional incarnations he had been a schoolteacher, farmer, editor, minister of the gospel, college president, and colonizer of the Louisiana Gulf Coast, where he had been the first man to introduce rice cultivation. Now, in

early 1906, he was three years into a new career that drew on all
the skills – pedagogical, agricultural, persuasive, evangelical, and
promotional – acquired over his first seven decades. As a special
agent for the Department of Agriculture, he had developed and
now ran the farm demonstration program, designed to help
Southern farmers get the most out of their land. Knapp's operational premise was the model of simplicity: "What a man hears he
may doubt. What he sees he may possibly doubt. But what he
does himself he cannot doubt."[34] Under the farm demonstration
program, Knapp would talk a group of local merchants and farmers into agreeing to indemnify one of their neighbors against
losses he might incur in the course of an experiment for which he
would volunteer. Under the terms of the agreement, he would cultivate one crop of cotton from seeds provided by the Department
of Agriculture and according to Knapp's instructions. One historian of the farm demonstration program has concluded that "the
indemnity fund . . . was important not because it was a financial
inducement to take a risk but because it was a social device which
psychologically ejected a remote authority whose praise or blame
was a matter of indifference, and replaced it with the vital and all-
important attention and opinion of one's lifelong friends and enemies."[35] Knapp himself explained why he thought the farm demonstration method worked so well. Once the local farmer had
agreed to Knapp's terms, the local paper would publish an article
describing the project and prominently mentioning the
volunteer's name. Knapp or one of his representatives would visit
the farm at least once a month to see how things were going and
would invite along anyone in the local area who was interested in
gauging the progress for himself.

Consequently he will almost unconsciously improve his farm so as to be
ready for company and cultivate all his crops better . . . A report of his
extra crop is made in the county papers. His neighbors talk about it and
want to buy seed . . . He sells the seed of his crop at a high price. His
neighbors ask him now he produced it. He is invited to address public as-
semblies. He has become a man of note and a leader of the people and
cannot return to his old ways. Soon there is a body of such men; a town-
ship, a county, and finally a State is transformed. The power which
transformed the humble fishermen of Galilee into mighty apostles of
truth is ever present and can be used as effectively today in any good
cause as when the Son of God turned His footsteps from Judea's capital
and spoke to the wayside children of poverty.[36]

The humble fishermen of Galilee, however, had not been scared
out of their wits by the boll weevil. Knapp's first experiments in

farm demonstration were carried out in 1903 in two northeastern Texas communities against a general backdrop of "panic and mass hysteria." The insect pest, which had crossed the Rio Grande a decade earlier, finally struck the Texas cotton crop with a vengeance that summer. The per-acre yield fell by 50 percent, and Texas cotton growers lost $15 million. Farmers threatened with impending doom were much more likely to become disciples of Knapp. Congress assisted the conversion process by appropriating $40,000 in late 1903 to extend the farm demonstration program into those Texas counties devastated the previous summer by the boll weevil. In 1904 over 7,000 farmers took up the "Knapp system," as it came to be called. As the menace continued its relentless eastward advance, so did Knapp's agents, winning over farmers in Louisiana and Arkansas by the score. The two early experiments in east Texas had both worked well enough, but Knapp owed the extraordinary immediate success of his system to the tenacity of the pest it was hoped he might obliterate. As it was, Knapp took Texas agriculture by storm. President Houston had introduced him to Buttrick as the other university in the state of Texas.[37]

After spending two days with Knapp going over the details of the farm demonstration system, Buttrick hurried back to New York where he reported to Gates that he had "been born again in Texas." Late in January 1906, Gates and Buttrick met in Washington with Knapp and Secretary of Agriculture James Wilson. No constitutional authority, Wilson informed them, would sanction the introduction of the demonstration program into states not yet ravaged by the boll weevil, but if the General Education Board would be generous enough to fund the work in areas still untouched, his department would cooperate in every other possible way. After the Board had appropriated an initial $7,000 for farm demonstration work in Mississippi, Buttrick and Wilson quietly signed an agreement whereby the Board contracted to send a monthly sum to Washington out of which the Department of Agriculture would pay a portion of Knapp's salary and those of the additional agents it could now hire to work in the uninfested parts of the South. As soon as the boll weevil turned up in a state, the agents there would become employees of the federal government in fact as well as on paper. In this manner, the General Education Board spent $925,750 between the spring of 1906 and the summer of 1914 in a slow and very quiet retreat along Sherman's old route – eastward through the Deep South to the sea, then northward to the Potomac.[38]

Under the clandestine patronage of the General Education Board, the Knapp system flourished. In fact, it grew and diversified in a way that it never would have had it remained exclusively dependent on government support. Congress had made the rapid expansion of Knapp's program possible in the first place, but only to combat the boll weevil. The Department of Agriculture would never have countenanced the speakers series, farm youth associations, financial counseling, and promotional literature that the General Education Board both encouraged and paid for. Gates himself was completely taken with Knapp personally and with his farm demonstration program. In his autobiography he called Knapp a genius and "a master of men as well. He knew the common farmer and he used his vast and minute knowledge in simple practical ways to multiply the farmer's net income by improved seed, better cultivation, diversification of crops, and accurate business methods in all departments of his household and farm life. I cannot undertake to describe here the boys' corn clubs or girls' canning clubs which he organized as side issues." Gates also grasped the significance of Knapp's appeal to his rural audiences. "I reflected that the farmer of the South leads a lonely and humdrum existence, craves variety and excitement, never misses a public gathering of any kind, is highly responsive to public appeal, and loves the political meeting and stump speaker, though the subject matter be very remotely, if indeed in any way at all connected with his private interests. What then might happen if speakers with due credentials should tell him facts of the highest personal consequence to himself?"[39]

Despite the depradations of the boll weevil, American agriculture flourished in the decade or so before the outbreak of the war in Europe. Richard Hofstadter has called it the "most prosperous period in modern times" for farmers. Southern farmers shared in the general prosperity to a lesser extent than did their counterparts in the farming regions of the Midwest and Pacific Coast states, but their lot did improve noticeably. Following as it did on the heels of a long agricultural depression and the aborted Populist uprising, the climb in farm prices must have lifted the spirits of rural Southerners and no doubt made them receptive to people like Knapp who told them how they could make even more. The generally improved economic situation also encouraged them to listen to the professors of secondary education and the state officers for primary instruction as well. Gates might possibly have known that his major Southern programs were launched at a time when Southern agriculture was more prosperous than it had been in anyone's memory, but he could hardly have foreseen that Southern farmers were not to enjoy such flush times again for another fifty years to come. When he first met Stiles in 1908, he did know that all his educational and demonstration programs were in place and working remarkably well. An indication, however, of the hidden assistance provided to the Rockefellers' Southern projects by impersonal market forces can be found in, of all places, the Depression legislation of the early 1930s establishing price levels for agricultural parities. The five years between 1909 and 1914 were chosen as the "base period" for farm programs. The same years marked the beginning and the end of the Rockefeller Sanitary Commission.[40]

# Two

# THE ROCKEFELLER
# SANITARY
# COMMISSION

# Wickliffe Rose Launches
# the Sanitary Commission

While Charles Wardell Stiles was wandering through the South in search of a patron, Gates was systematically constructing, with Rockefeller's money, a philanthropic empire in medical research and public education. It remained for the two men to be introduced. Their eventual encounter represented the culmination of a sequence of events that began with a series of informal conversations between Stiles and Walter Hines Page, brought together on the same train by Theodore Roosevelt for a completely different reason. Page, a North Carolinian by birth and a well-known "professional Southerner" by choice despite years of exile in New York as a magazine editor and publisher, came to know Stiles well in 1908 while both men were serving on the President's Commission on Country Life.

Called "the great galvanizing event in the history of the rural reform movement of the early twentieth century,"[1] the Commission was summoned into existence by Roosevelt in August 1908, amid considerable national publicity, "to investigate the economic, social, and sanitary conditions of country life throughout the United States."[2] That it actually accomplished anything of value is remarkable, since the Commission spent its brief life almost entirely in the shadow of presidential politics. The announcement of its creation came from the White House shortly after the Democratic Convention had once again nominated the self-styled friend of country folk throughout the United States, William Jennings Bryan. And, by calling for its final report no later than January 1, 1909, Roosevelt ensured that he, not one of his two possible successors, would be sitting behind the President's desk to receive it. Blue ribbon presidential commissions, he well knew, were notorious for exceeding their allotted spans, but a gap of almost four months between the publicized expiration date and the upcoming inauguration would surely guarantee that, the vagaries of national elections notwithstanding, a Republican would be there to reap the benefits of this Republican initiative.[3]

With the life expectancy, then, of a bubble on the roiling surface of American presidential politics, the Country Life Commission could not afford the luxury of a thorough, methodical investigation. Its members – all prominent academicians, journalists, and high-ranking government officials[4] – quickly adopted out of necessity a rather impressionistic, four-phase program for gathering information. They began by enlisting the cooperation of two agencies of the federal government. The Post Office delivered over 500,000 questionnaires to farmers living on rural free delivery routes, and the Census Bureau tabulated and analyzed close to 100,000 of the approximately 115,000 responses by the time the Commission's final report went to the printers. The President himself issued a strongly worded appeal to farmers across the country to meet in district schools and discuss the issues raised by twelve questions on the circulars. Reports from about 200 of these meetings in 36 states had reached the Commission's office before it closed its doors. Each member of the Commission pursued, in addition, a special line of investigation on his own and prepared his findings for inclusion in the final report. Lastly, the Commission, sitting as a group, held public hearings in thirty places across the country.[5]

It was while touring the South with the Commission that Stiles and Page struck up an acquaintance. When Stiles had read of Roosevelt's new organization to investigate country living he saw it as another opportunity to lobby for his favorite cause. He turned to William H. Welch to intercede with the President on his behalf. Welch had known Stiles since 1897, when the zoologist first began lecturing occasionally at Johns Hopkins. Welch too had studied for a time in Leipzig, where Leuckart's lectures had removed the last shreds of doubt in his mind regarding the probability of natural selection. As the editor of the *Journal of Experimental Medicine*, he had drawn on Stiles's vast knowledge of scientific nomenclature. He therefore willingly approached Roosevelt with Stiles's request. Shortly thereafter, Stiles received an invitation to join the Country Life Commission as its medical attaché.[6]

Page had missed the Commission's earlier tours of the Midwest and Pacific Coast but was along in November 1908 for the trip through the South. Early one morning, he, Stiles, and a third member of the Commission, Henry Wallace – "Uncle Henry" to the rural readers of his Des Moines journal, *Wallace's Farmer*, and the father and grandfather of future secretaries of agriculture – sat talking in the smoking car. While waiting to complete a stop at a small country station between Goldsboro and Raleigh, Wallace noted and commented on the unfortunate appearance of one of the men lounging about on the station platform. Stiles later remembered him for Mark Sullivan as a

type hardly to be recognized as human, misshapen, his dwarfish body small in proportion to his apparently elongated limbs and fingers and unnaturally swollen joints; shoulders hunched and pointed, neck attenuated like that of a very old man, his dropsically protuberant stomach forming a hideous contrast with his pathetically emaciated unnourished frame; skin the greenish-yellow tint of tallow, shrivelled and parchment-like, eyes like a fragment of faded rag, nose almost transparent, mouth sagging; his attitude, that of a three-fourths empty sack supported by contact with the station wall.[7]

This wretch was a representative of a class of Southerners all too familiar to Page. He explained to Wallace, who had never encountered such a pitiful creature in the robust Iowa farm regions, that the man was a "dirt-eater," one of the more depressing elements in the South's chronic farm labor problem.[8]

At this point Stiles spoke up. The farmer's condition, he said, was due to severe hookworm infection. With fifty cents' worth of drugs and a few weeks' rest he could be completely cured. Page, always receptive to a scheme that might somehow lead to the regeneration of the South, listened attentively while Stiles explained the extent to which this parasite had undermined human health in his native region. Untold numbers of Southerners – men, women, and children of both races and from every social and economic niche – were leading miserable, unproductive lives as a direct result of the hookworm's ravages. Stiles also mentioned that for the past six years he had been saying much the same thing to anyone who would listen, but that few were both willing and in a position to do anything about it.

When the Commissioners' train reached Raleigh, the members held a public hearing at which Stiles, with Page's encouragement, estimated that fully 35 percent of North Carolina's schoolchildren were anemic because of hookworm disease. Governor Robert B. Glenn and Josephus Daniels, editor of the *Raleigh News and Observer* and later to become Wilson's Secretary of the Navy, were scandalized. "I am not at all pleased with the character of the talks made," fumed the governor, "as they had more of the appearance of being an attempt to injure the State than to improve it. I do not believe that the coming of such a commission tends to do any good when the statements made by them are in direct conflict with true conditions."[9] The *News and Observer* berated Page for countenancing slander directed at the land of his birth and published sketches of his father and grandfather, both of whom lived to ripe old ages, to prove that nowhere in the land were the people healthier than in North Carolina. Page, grown accustomed over the years to just such a reaction whenever he suggested that conditions at home were less than ideal, stood his ground and remained unshaken in his support of Stiles.[10]

Eight days later, while still on the Southern tour, Page and Stiles routinely left the train for a few minutes to buy the daily newspapers. A certain front page article sent Stiles into an immediate and profound depression which, by his own account, left him almost speechless for several days. Page, who worried for his friend's health, eventually pried the truth from him. It seemed that after years of bad luck, Stiles had finally struck it rich a few weeks earlier. A friend had approached him in his Washington club with the news that a wealthy Southerner wished to donate $2 million toward a plan to improve the South. He had attached two conditions: that his gift be made anonymously, and that it go to a cause still undiscovered by any other philanthropist. Stiles got in touch with the man and persuaded him that his money would best be spent underwriting an attempt to purge his region of hookworm disease. The benefactor agreed and authorized Stiles to select a board of trustees and to devise a plan of operation. Stiles, who for years had been hoping for such a windfall, was not long at his assignment. His tentative board included Dr. Welch and Surgeon-General Wyman. When he had left Washington with the Country Life Commission for the Southern trip, he had expected the announcement of the gift within two weeks, but now the newspapers told of his would-be angel's sudden death. He had not signed the agreement.

Stiles had sworn never to reveal the man's identity in connection with the donation, and even though the plan collapsed, he scrupulously kept the secret for the rest of his life, except to mention the incident without names in his autobiographical account of the early days of the hookworm campaign. In all likelihood, however, the man whom Stiles mourned that Saturday morning on a Southern railroad platform was Joseph Bryan of Richmond, one of the wealthiest men in the South and a philanthropist of some note, and one who would not have turned a hair at the re-criminations leveled at Stiles by the anti-child-labor people. An especially noteworthy member of a distinctive caste of nine-teenth-century Southerners, any one of whom might well have served as the prototype of Colonel John Sartoris if Faulkner had not found one on his own family tree, Bryan had simply redirec-ted the conspicuous resources of cunning and tenacity that had served him well as a young cavalryman to build a business empire out of the meager legacy of Appomattox. His youthful predilec-tion for killing Yankees, destroying trains, and tearing up rail-road tracks did not preclude his ready acceptance, after the shooting had stopped, of Yankee business practices and Yankee business partners to build new trains and finance miles of new tracks. At the time of his death, Bryan owned the Richmond Lo-comotive Works and a controlling interest in the *Richmond Times-Dispatch*. He sat on the board of directors of several pre-dominantly Southern companies, among them the Southern Rail-way, the Equitable Life Assurancy Society, the Sloss-Sheffield Company, and the North Birmingham Land Company. A consci-entious son of the Old Dominion as well, Bryan, according to his obituary notice in the *Washington Post*, "was recognized as one of the South's greatest philanthropists who never allowed an op-portunity for advancing Southern interests to escape him."[11] At the age of sixty-two he died of heart trouble following a very brief and unexpected illness. Stiles read of his passing on Saturday, November 21, 1908.

Though Stiles left Bryan's name out of his narrative, Page (who also kept the secret) had little difficulty guessing his identity. In an effort to reassure the crestfallen scientist who must have thought that his hookworm program was never to be, Page men-tioned that Bryan was not the only man in the country with the means and the inclination to finance programs to better the South. The remark was made in passing, and nothing immedi-ately came of it, but Page had a man in mind.

After completing the Southern tour, the members of the Coun-try Life Commission journeyed to Ithaca, New York, for their final public hearing and a reception in their honor on the campus of Cornell University. Liberty Hyde Bailey, the chairman of the Commission, was the dean of the College of Agriculture at Cor-nell. In the course of the evening, Stiles was approached by a plump, friendly-looking man who introduced himself as Wallace Buttrick, a friend of Page's who had been asked by the journalist to seek Stiles out at his earliest convenience and hear what he had to say. Buttrick, as it happened, lived close to Page on Teaneck Road in Englewood, New Jersey. Page, of course, was an active member of Buttrick's General Education Board, but he had other ties to the Rockefellers as well. Most recently, he had serialized the senior John D. Rockefeller's "Random Reminiscences" in his own magazine, *World's Work*, at a time when the Rockefeller name was receiving almost daily publicity of a more lurid kind during another state legislative committee investigation of Standard Oil. Page had followed up on his hint to Stiles by getting in touch with Buttrick upon his return to New York. Stiles left the reception with the emissary of the Rockefeller philanthropies and returned to Buttrick's hotel room where, according to one account, they "talked hookworm almost all night." Nothing definite sprang from their first meeting, but Buttrick did promise to relay Stiles's information to his associates in New York.[12]

While Stiles returned to the Hygienic Laboratory in Washington, Buttrick went immediately to Gates with his news. Gates, who later claimed to have remembered the original *New York Sun* article, listened carefully to the account of Buttrick's meeting with Stiles. "My imagination," he later wrote, "began to play around the alleged devastation and suffering caused by this disease."[13] But to the wary Gates, the important word in that sentence was "alleged." He conferred with Simon Flexner, who had known Stiles at Johns Hopkins and could vouch for his integrity and scientific attainments. Flexner also gave his considerable support to Stiles's theory. A telegram from Flexner brought Stiles north again, this time for a formal demonstration in Gates's office. His presentation burnished to a high luster by years of practice, Stiles arrived with specimen case, microscope, drawings, photographs, lantern slides, and statistics—all the arcana of his obsession. After listening for about forty minutes, Gates interrupted to call Starr J. Murphy, Rockefeller's personal attorney. When Murphy arrived, Gates said, "This is the biggest proposition ever put to the Rockefeller Office. Now, Doctor, start from the beginning and tell Mr. Murphy what you have told me."[14] Gates heard him out in silence this time before turning to the more practical questions of program and finance. He was taken somewhat aback to learn that Stiles had no precise answers to some of the larger questions. Perhaps there were as many as two million hookworm victims in the Southern states, but since no survey had been conducted no one could say with any degree of assurance. Despite his mounting enthusiasm, Gates decided the matter required more investigation. Stiles returned to Washington without a commitment from Rockefeller's lieutenants, or even a promise that the matter would be taken up with Rockefeller himself. But Gates did encourage Stiles to look more thoroughly into the broader demographic aspects of the hookworm problem.[15]

Gates and Murphy, in the meantime, undertook with Flexner's assistance an investigation of their own. They solicited the views of physicians, educators, and public men throughout the South. Stiles may not have made much headway at the grass-roots level, but he had persuaded a few men at the top. Gates also looked closely at Ashford's work in Puerto Rico and at the reasons behind the Florida Board of Health's recent decision to move against hookworm on its own initiative. The results of Gates's research bore out Stiles's predictions; indeed, they went the zoologist one better. "These studies," wrote Gates, "consumed much valuable time, but . . . his estimate of two million cases was not exaggerated. It proved in the sequel to be an understatement." The fact that Stiles had initially underestimated the size of the problem must have struck the cautious Gates as an indication of a salutary prudence in the scientist's character, a check on his obvious zeal. In any event, he continued: "I was now ready to present the matter to the Messrs. Rockefeller, Senior and Junior. They recognized the high importance of the subject and committed themselves to the needed funds for a campaign of extermination of the hookworm in the United States."[16] The use of the word "extermination" in more public contexts would eventually return to haunt Gates and the others.

With the consent of the Rockefellers firmly established, Gates turned privately to tactical considerations. "The South was still sensitive and angry. We could do nothing effective without cordial Southern cooperation. A board of distinguished and influential Southern men must be organized. I could easily name such a board, but would they accept membership in the face of a hostile South? I made a tentative list of the men we needed, and made my plans for enlisting them." Two such lists, both containing many of the same names, were readily to hand. One consisted of members of the General Education Board; the other, of directors of its predecessor and close institutional partner, the Southern Education Board. "Fortunately there was about to be held at the hospitable mansion of Mr. George Peabody, at Lake George, a conference on Southern Education, to be attended by most of the very men on my list." Stiles, still on tenterhooks eight months after his initial meeting with Gates, was summoned to Lake

George. "It was easy," Gates continued, "to persuade Mr. Peabody to set aside an evening for the stereopticon lecture of Dr. Stiles. The evening came and the effect was overwhelming. The Southern guests immediately recognized the mysterious 'ground itch' of their barefoot boyhood." After the demonstration, Gates announced that the Rockefeller office would support the work. Before the guests had retired for the evening, he had formed his board.

A few weeks later, Gates invited Stiles to spend the night in Montclair and to discuss the details of the upcoming campaign. The two men's accounts of their meeting vary widely on certain points under discussion that evening. Stiles recalled that Gates first proposed the sum of $50,000 for the project. Such a small amount would, in Stiles's opinion, barely cover the initial stages of organization. One million dollars represented a far more realistic estimate. In Gates's account, the final sum is the same, but it was reached in an altogether different manner. "Dr. Stiles had thought half a million dollars would be needed, and this Mr. Rockefeller had promised me before the Lake George meeting. But to startle the South we fixed on a million, with Mr. Rockefeller's consent."[17] Stiles also recalled that Gates agreed to the higher figure only on the condition that Stiles resign from government service and devote all his time to directing the campaign. Gates's autobiography mentions the discussion of Stiles's resignation but no offer of the directorship; on this subject it remains studiously silent. Stiles remembered being reluctant to leave his post in Washington. "I explained to him that I thought I could present a better plan and that I would give him my answer in the morning."[18]

The next day, Stiles handed Gates a letter of resignation addressed to Surgeon-General Wyman, but asked that it not be mailed until after Stiles had been given at least forty-eight hours notice by telegram. One latter-day student of these negotiations has contented that the letter was a gambit on Stiles's part. If one accepts Stiles's version of the meeting, this conclusion seems reasonable. By acceding, at least for the moment, to Gates's single stipulation of his resignation, Stiles could counter with a proposal of his own on the organization of the campaign. In his opinion, the Sanitary Commission would face its biggest and most important challenge in the rural schools. Very few of them had privies of any sort; few teachers were yet aware that the lack of sanitary facilities posed a threat to health. If Rockefeller's gift were dropped into the pond at this strategic point, the ripples would

reach and transform the most remote corners of Southern society
in a very short time. In order to enlist the active cooperation of
teachers and students across the South, however, the educational
hierarchy must be first won over. Stiles believed the best way to
convert the leaders of the Southern schools would be by appoint-
ing one of their own to administer the campaign. He suggested J.
Y. Joyner of North Carolina, state superintendent of schools and
one of the few Southerners in a position of public authority who
had listened seriously to Stiles in the past.[19]

For the better part of a decade Joyner had been caught up in
the fight of his professional life with the North Carolina legislature over the issue of free public schools. He had been appointed
to his post in 1902 by Governor Charles B. Aycock, known na-
tionally for his twin beliefs in white supremacy and free public education. Stiles had managed to persuade Joyner privately that
hookworm disease sabotaged his educational system just as
surely as any assemblage of antediluvian politicians, but Joyner,
reluctant to dissipate his energy and influence on more than one
issue, had not acted on his new conviction. Aycock was gone, and
his successor, Governor Glenn, had made his views on the subject
of hookworm disease quite clear following the Country Life Commission's public hearing in Raleigh.[20]

Stiles also later claimed that he intimated to Gates that Surgeon-General Wyman might be induced to assign a cadre of Public Health Service officers with Southern backgrounds to work
through the state boards of health with local physicians and educators. The federal government would continue to pay their salaries, but the Rockefellers could pick up their expenses. Stiles remembered arguing that his own talents would best be employed,
not in administration, but in the same old ways — research and
public lectures before medical schools, universities, and service
groups. By remaining in government service and by joining in the
work with a group of fellow health officers, he could bring the
prestige and influence of the national government into an alliance
with their privately funded effort. At the same time, he would
pre-empt with one stroke those who might be tempted to suggest
that, having failed to convince the government of the importance
of the work, he had turned in desperation to a gullible millionaire.[21]

Though certainly not gullible, Rockefeller's philanthropic directors had proved far more receptive to Stiles's proposal than any
of his superiors, save Wyman, in the federal bureaucracy. His inability to shake funds and assistants out of the Treasury Depart-

ment had forced him to look for private sources of revenue. Stiles must also have sensed that the name Rockefeller was not the talisman to bring about a favorable change of heart in Roosevelt's administration. If his letter of resignation was just a feint, then, in a small battle of wills with Gates, Stiles had squandered part of the opportunity it brought on a proposal that both he and Gates must have known was far-fetched.

Though his is the most comprehensive version of this important *tête-à-tête* with Gates, Stiles's account must not be taken completely at face value. He wrote it in 1939, after Gates, Buttrick, Page, and Rockefeller, Sr. – the other men who might possibly have been a part of the discussions leading to a choice of directors and might have been in a position to challenge his recollection of the facts – had all died without leaving, as far as he knew, any contradictory reports. Stiles was unaware of Gates's private autobiography, but even had it been available to him when he was writing his own article, it would not have forced him to question his memory on that key question. Gates's journal does go on at some length to present a completely different record of the negotiations regarding the new organization's finances, but nowhere does it mention that Stiles had been offered, and declined, the directorship. Why would Stiles, assuming that the job of chief administrative officer had been his for the taking as he later said it was, suddenly balk at the opportunity to manage a campaign that he had been working incessantly for seven years to bring about? His friends purportedly thought him miffed that someone else was selected.[22]

Gates may well have decided on his own that Stiles was unsuited for the position and, as a result, never have offered it to him. Stiles had no administrative experience to speak of, and furthermore anyone who knew him as well as Gates did by this time knew him to be a rather prickly character, not the sort whom one might confidently expect to work smoothly with a large staff of employees or to maneuver deftly around countless Southern doctors, editors, and politicians. Nor had his old nemesis, the anti-child-labor lobby, entirely forgotten him either. In a letter to Simon Flexner after the public announcement of the Commission's formation, Lillian Wald of the Henry Street Settlement warned that Stiles would drive away many who might otherwise rally to the support of the new organization. Gates himself wrote in a letter to the man who would eventually take the administrative secretary's post, "The only opposition which I really fear is the opposition on the parts of the opponents of child labor who

who are thoroughly organized and also the opposition of organized labor, and that has been due to their misunderstanding of
Dr. Stiles."[23] Rockefeller himself generated more than enough
controversy; from Stiles and from his own investigations Gates
had come to learn the very idea of hookworm disease was also
capable of provoking strong feelings. The fledgling Sanitary
Commission would have to live with the reputation of its patron,
and it could do very little at the outset about the popularity of its
target, but it need not compound two controversies with a third.
For whatever reasons, Stiles was not charged with the responsibilities of overseeing the daily activities of the program he had
done so much to create. At its first official meeting, the Rockefeller Sanitary Commission for the Eradication of Hookworm
Disease firmly resolved that the "question of child labor is not related in any way to the purposes or work of this commission."[24]
Although they had not been able to drive him out of the Public
Health Service the year before, there is good reason to believe
that the anti-child-labor people had played a large part in block-
ing Stiles from the one job he wanted above all others.

Gates took two months to put the finishing touches on his arrangements for launching the Commission. On October 26, 1909,
John D. Rockefeller, Sr. addressed a letter (probably drafted by
Gates, or at least with his assistance) to the twelve men who had
agreed to serve on the executive committee. He promised to put
$1 million at their disposal over a five-year period and outlined
his reasons for undertaking the work.

Gentlemen:
    For many months my representatives have been inquiring into the na-
ture and prevalence of "Hookworm Disease," and considered plans for
mitigating its evils. I have delayed action in this matter only until the
facts as to the extent of the disease could be verified and the effectiveness of its cure and prevention demonstrated. The wide distribution and
serious effects of this malady, particularly in the rural districts of our
Southern states, first pointed out by Dr. Charles Wardell Stiles of the
United States Public Health and Marine-Hospital Sevice, have been confirmed by independent investigators and physicians, as well as by educators, and public men in the South.
    Knowing your interest in all that pertains to the well-being of your fel-
low men and your acquaintance with this subject, I have invited you to a
conference in the hope that it may lead to the adoption of well-considered
plans for a co-operative movement of the Medical Profession, Public
Health Officials, Board of Trade, Churches, Schools, the Press, and other
agencies, for the cure and prevention of this disease. If you deem it wise
to undertake this commission, I shall be glad to be permitted to work

with you to that end and you may call upon me from time to time for such sums as may be needed during the next five years for carrying on an aggressive campaign, up to a total of one million dollars ($1,000,000).

While it would be a privilege to act in any movement which offers assurance of relieving human suffering, it is also a peculiar pleasure to me to feel that the principal activities of your Board will be among the people of our Southern States. It has been my pleasure of late to spend a portion of each year in the South and I have come to know and to respect greatly that part of our country and to enjoy the society and friendship of many of its warm-hearted people. It will therefore be an added gratification to me if in this way I may in some measure express my appreciation of their kindnesses and hospitalities.[25]

The ten men assembled in New York in anticipation of Rockefeller's announcement[26] were quick to respond. In their reply, also dated October 26, 1909, they thanked him for the "opportunity to be of service to [their] fellow men" and accepted his "invitation to administer this trust."[27]

Included on the Commission's first board of directors were eight men already involved in the work of either the Institute for Medical Research or the General Education Board. They were Welch, now the president of the American Medical Association, Flexner, Gates, Murphy, Alderman, Frissell, Page, and Rockefeller, Jr. Three men—Joyner of North Carolina, P. P. Claxton, Professor of Education at the University of Tennessee, and David F. Houston, the man who had first introduced Buttrick to Knapp and who had since become chancellor of Washington University in St. Louis—were new to the management of the Rockefeller philanthropies but had worked closely with the General Education Board in the past. Stiles, at whose emotions on the occasion one can only guess, rounded out the board of directors. Of the total of twelve, three were doctors or scientists, three were from the Rockefeller offices, one was a journalist, and five were educators.

The irrepressible Page left no doubt regarding his own feelings at the time. Later in the evening of the same day he jubilantly noted:

The Rockefeller Commission for the Extermination of the Hookworm Disease: To-day this organization was made, with the gift of a million dollars by John D. Rockefeller . . . The one greatest single cause of anaemia and stagnation in the South will by this fund be ultimately removed, and 2,000,000 inefficient people be made well.

This result came about from the work of the Country Life Commission appointed by President Roosevelt, and from my bringing Dr. Stiles within the range of Dr. Buttrick's and Mr. Gates's knowledge and interest.

It is the largest single benefit that could be done to the people of the South. This is one of the inheritances of slavery, the disease having been brought by Negroes.

A very big day's work indeed.

A big day's work for the old land![28]

Page had loosely used the word "extermination" in the hastily chosen title he unofficially gave the new organization, and he predicted that hookworm disease would be "utlimately removed" from the Southern landscape. Rockefeller, on the other hand, had been much more circumspect in his letter. Avoiding a call for a final solution to the hookworm problem, he had urged instead that the Commission's directors pledge themselves to the far more modest goal of finding ways to mitigate the disease's evils. Stiles later claimed to have cautioned Gates and the others that hookworm disease would prove to be much more intractable than they, in the first flush of enthusiasm, had anticipated. It would take the allotted five-year life span of the Commission just to begin to move in the right direction, he warned, and talk of "extermination" or "eradication" would be inappropriate for at least another generation. Gates, not oblivious to the medical niceties of Stiles's argument, chose to pursue a goal other than strict scientific accuracy when he decided to include the word "eradication" in the Commission's official title. To achieve any degree of success the Commission would have to challenge the imaginations and galvanize the energies of thousands of Southerners, most of whom would be more likely to lend their support to something billed in advance as a pitched battle rather than a protracted war of attrition. Southerners, after all, had always been historically predisposed more toward the lightning calvary charge than the siege of indefinite duration.

The name "Sanitary Commission" had an illustrious history of its own. It had come to signify a paramilitary organization called into existence to meet a specific crisis and disbanded once its purposes had been met. The British Sanitary Commission had tended the sick and wounded in the Crimean War. Florence Nightingale had worked under its auspices. Closer to home, the United States Sanitary Commission had served the same purpose for the Union armies during the Civil War. With Lincoln's approval the civilians who staffed and administered the U.S. Sanitary Commission strove, in the words of George M. Fredrickson, "to revise the American system of values as [well as] to relieve the suffering of the wounded," and they saw their work "as a heaven sent opportunity for educating the nation."[29] The five academic figures on the Rockefeller Sanitary Commission's board of directors, along with Gates and the others from the General Education Board, likewise conceived of their work in educational terms, although their smaller and more immediate purpose, like that of the U.S. Sanitary Commission fifty years earlier, was a medical one. The U.S. Sanitary Commission had exercised a strong influence on the course of American philanthropy after the Civil War, an impact that Fredrickson has called conservative and has located in the "belief in the need for an expert to act as intermediary between irrational popular benevolence and the suffering to be relieved."[30] The leaders of the U.S. Sanitary Commission, from the upper ranks of mid-nineteenth-century Northern society, had been striving to reassert a kind of social control over their less wellborn fellow citizens through the imposition of order and discipline in the amelioration of suffering. Gates and his associates, good progressives all, believed no less strongly in the need for an elite of professional experts, not social betters. The Rockefeller Sanitary Commissioners were certainly aware of the accomplishments of the U.S. Sanitary Commission; they could not have been blind to the connotations of the name they adopted for their own organization.

In the two months immediately following the October meeting, Gates saw to the drafting of a set of by-laws, modeled on the structural format of the General Education Board, which set forth the official purpose of the Commission. Taken almost verbatim from Rockefeller's letter, the statement of purpose bound the Commission "to bring about a cooperative movement of the medical profession, public health officials, boards of trade, churches, schools, the press and other agencies for the cure and prevention of hookworm disease." Gates also made sure that the broader objectives of the Commission were given expression in its by-laws: "While pursuing its own definite object — the eradication of hookworm disease — it would seek to conduct its work in such a way as to stimulate and guide state and local efforts in building up in each state a system of permanent agencies which would take care of the whole problem of public health."[31]

As was the custom in such documents, the Commission's by-laws also established a regular time for annual meetings and called for the selection of a slate of officers to guide the work. Since over half of the members of the Commission's board of directors would already have to come to New York for the annual meeting of the General Education Board in January, Gates decided to schedule the meetings of the Rockefeller Sanitary Commission to coincide. He became the chairman of the Commission, a position whose holder (according to the job description he wrote himself) would be required to "sustain an executive and advisory relation to the work and policies of the Commission similar to that usually sustained by the chairman or president of commercial bodies."[32] Gates who remained as chairman throughout the five years of the Commission's existence, did not play an active, day-to-day part in the work, but he did preside over board meetings and exercised a profound influence over the direction that work took. L. G. Myers, a businessman who had managed the accounts of some of the Rockefeller philanthropies in the past, became the Commission's treasurer. As in the case of the chairman, Myers's duties as custodian of the funds and securities of the Commission were no different from those of the treasurer of any business enterprise. Like Gates, Myers retained his position for the duration of the Commission's activities.

The problem persisted of what to do with Stiles. The zoologist was indeed turning out to be something of a nuisance. Without waiting for Gates's approval, he had approached Surgeon-General Wyman with the plan he had outlined to Gates in Montclair. Wyman had tentatively agreed to Stiles's proposal once he determined that it would be based on the precedent established by Buttrick and Secretary of Agriculture Wilson. He was prepared to place at the disposal of the state boards of health a group of Public Health Service officers, all born in the South, to assist in the work of hookworm eradication. As with Knapp's agents in the states already hit by the boll weevil, the government would pay their salaries while the Sanitary Commission would pick up all their expenses. The Secretary of the Treasury – Wyman's boss – would have none of it, however. He would only consent to give Stiles a one-year leave of absence without pay to work for the Sanitary Commission. As Stiles later grumbled, "Had the plan been approved, the entire scheme, since adopted, of cooperation between boards of health and the U.S. Public Health Service would have been put into immediate effect."[33]

Rather than place any administrative responsibility in Stiles's hands, Gates resorted to a Solomon-like expedient. He cut off a small portion of what would otherwise have fallen to the lot of the administrative secretary – the Commission's equivalent to Buttrick – and gave those duties, complete with the title of scientific secretary, to Stiles. As befitted his stature as the John the Baptist of the hookworm work, Stiles would be more involved in the mundane routine essential to the Commission's proper functioning than either Gates or Myers but in such a way that the potential damage he might do to the public relations effort of the other Rockefeller people would be minimized in advance. He would remain in the Public Health Service, and when his duties there permitted he would represent the Commission "before scientific and other bodies, and in addresses to and work with members of the medical profession."[34] In short, Stiles was ultimately responsible for the medical and scientific aspects of the work, but as both he and Gates knew, those aspects would be clearly subordinate to the educational and promotional ones. It is a tribute to Stiles's tenacity that he was able to make as much of his position as he did, for it would seem that Gates had intended it to be little more than ceremonial.

The job of the Commission's principal *chargé d'affaires* would fall to the administrative secretary. Joyner was everyone's first choice to fill this, the most important of the Commission's offices. He had been unable to make the trip to New York in October to be on hand to receive Rockefeller's letter, but he had let the participants know that he would gladly serve on the board of directors. A meeting in Chicago of the National Educational Association, of which he was president, had conflicted with the Rockefeller announcement, and it was there that Page reached him by telegram to urge to stop in New York on his way back to North Carolina. Page met him at the train station and began the three days of intensive pressure designed to make Joyner accept the post. He was whisked away to a luncheon meeting with Rockefeller, Jr., Gates, Buttrick, and others, after which he accompanied Gates home to Montclair to find Stiles waiting for him. The next day, Buttrick guided him through the offices of the General Education Board to a room next to Buttrick's own office, affording an excellent panorama of the harbor, and announced that it would be Joyner's if he saw fit to accept Gates's offer. Joyner, who seems to have been somewhat bemused by the suggestion, is supposed to have answered, "I am not the first man to be taken to a high place and offered the world."[35] He left New York without giving Gates a decision and returned to North Carolina by way of Charlottesville, where he stopped long enough to confer with Alderman.

Once back in Raleigh, far away from the temptations of New York and up to his neck again in his local concerns, Joyner decided to reject the offer.

It seems clear to me . . . that it would be a blunder for me to sever my official connection with the educational forces of the State and the South to be the paid Administrative Secretary of the Rockefeller Commission, for I am convinced that I would thereby greatly decrease my ability to aid effectively in the organization of these forces into active and enthusiastic support of the movement for the eradication of the hookworm disease, that I can exert more influence in securing the cooperation of all other classes of my people in the successful prosecution of this important work as their respresentative, laboring without compensation from other sources, and therefore, without suspicion of other motive than an unselfish desire to serve them in a great public health movement, most intimately related to the work to which they have called me and for which they are paying me.

In the final analysis, Joyner felt he could "be of more service as Superintendent of Public Instruction and as the representative of all my people."[36] Reading between the carefully worded lines of Joyner's letter, it was clear that he was loath to abandon his struggle for free public schools in North Carolina in order to take on a job for which he really did not feel qualified. It was too far outside his line of work.

Joyner had taken several weeks to make up his mind, and it was now late in the fall of 1909. Someone would have to be found to head the Commission, and quickly, too, if it was to open its doors for business with the new year, as Gates hoped. Under the by-laws, the administrative secretary's tasks would include all facets of the Commission's activities not specifically assigned to another officer. Of the four executive officers, he would be the only full-time one. Clearly, an inept administrative secretary would seriously jeopardize the success of the whole venture.

In December 1909, Gates offered the job for the the second time, and again to a professional educator. Wickliffe Rose (1862-1931) — Dean of George Peabody College and the University of Nashville, General Agent of the Peabody Fund, Executive Secretary of the Southern Education Board, and member of the Slater Fund — was already known to the educators on the Commission's board of directors. Page, who made a point of knowing every Southerner with progressive leanings in a position of authority, also thought highly of Rose. So did Buttrick, who first called him to Gates's attention after Joyner's decision.

Forty-seven years old when he first met Gates, Rose, like Joyner, had certainly not been preparing all his life for such an offer and was caught completely unawares when it came. In fact, it is unclear whether he had even heard of hookworm disease before he read in the papers of Rockefeller's gift to combat it. Now, barely a month later, he had been invited to abandon his old career and immediately assume control of the program to bring about the eradication of hookworm disease. From all appearances, he was a most improbable candidate for the job. He certainly thought so. His first reaction was one of bewilderment, as if Gates had made a mistake and confused him with someone else. When he recovered from his initial shock, he came very close to turning Gates down out of hand. Gates, who may have learned something about courting and winning educators from his recent experience with Joyner, urged Rose to take his time and think it over before rushing headlong into a decision.[37]

By all accounts, it was a difficult decision to make. Simon Flexner recalled that he happened to be at Lake George when Rose was there for a meeting of the Southern Education Board. The two men rowed out into the lake one evening—this, in December—while Rose spoke in anguished tones of his dilemma. Later, he told Raymond Fosdick that he could not sleep properly until after he had made up his mind. When he finally did accept, it was with the assurances of Gates and the others that the work would not stop with hookworm disease even though the Sanitary Commission was to be funded for only five years. On January 15, 1910, at the first annual meeting of the directors of the Sanitary Commission, Page placed Rose's name in nomination for the position of administrative secretary at a salary of $7,500 per year plus expenses, "with the understanding that he is to remain without salary as the Secretary of the Peabody and Southern Education Boards but is to turn over most of his work to his subordinates."[38] Rose had decided that he could not leave his colleagues in Nashville completely in the lurch, although the demand of the Sanitary Commission would leave him practically no time to give to the Peabody merger. In the meantime, he had not waited for the Commission's directors to make his appointment official. Less than a month after his acceptance he moved to Washington, where on January 8, 1910, he opened an office in the Union Trust Building. He and Gates had agreed that an official headquarters south of the Mason-Dixon line but in the neutral District of Columbia would help to soften the Commission's carpetbagger image. Stiles's base of operations was not far away—on the corner of 24th and E Streets, N.W.[39]

Wickliffe Rose, as it turned out, was an excellent choice for the job despite his self-admitted ignorance of public health matters.

He had been born in rural Tennessee, in Saulsbury, on November 19, 1862, during the thick of the fight in the border states. Until he was well into his twenties, Rose divided his time between his father's harvests: of cotton on the family farm and souls in the local Disciples of Christ church, where the elder Rose preached the fundamentalist gospel to the Hardeman County faithful for half a century. It took a chance reading of Plato to spirit young Rose away to Nashville. "The elegant idealism of the dialogues transported me into a new existence in another world," he later wrote. "Here began my intellectual life."[40] Under the spell of the classical Greeks he enrolled at the University of Nashville in the mid-1880s.[41]

The school had fallen on hard times after the Civil War, but had avoided disaster by combining with the new State Normal College in 1875 under a merger arrangement worked out and financed by the Peabody Fund. Rose took his bachelor's degree in 1889, the year before the school's name was changed to the Peabody Normal College and University of Nashville. This second administrative shuffle accounts for the confusing fact that even though Rose took an M.A. degree in 1890 from the same school that awarded him his B.A., the names of the degree-granting institutions were different. Rose maintained his enthusiasm for the ancients while in college, choosing to concentrate in Greek Education with minors in political philosophy and French. His master's thesis was an analysis of Plato's *Republic*. He stayed on at his alma mater after his graduation to take a position as Instructor in History and Mathematics, and after a year he was made a full professor. For the next ten years he taught history and the philosophy of education and worked to build up an endowment for the financially troubled school. He left in 1902 to accept a post in philosophy at the University of Tennessee at Knoxville but returned two years later to take up new duties as dean of both the Peabody Normal College and the University of Nashville. Finding the two schools still beset with money problems, he entered into negotiations with the representatives of the Peabody Fund to find a way to solve their financial difficulties once and for all. An agreement was reached whereby the trustees of the Peabody Fund would gradually wind up their affairs and transfer the funds under their control into the endowment of the two Nashville colleges. For their part, the Peabody Normal College and the University of Nashville would submerge their separate identities into a single new institution to be called the George Peabody College for Teachers. The administrators of the Peabody Fund had decided that their small philanthropy had recently been eclipsed by much larger organizations like the General Education Board. The Nashville merger gave them an opportunity to phase the Fund out of existence. In 1907, Rose resigned his deanship to become the General Agent of the Peabody Fund, to preside over its liquidation and oversee the transition in Nashville. When Gates invited him to come to New York to discuss the Rockefeller Sanitary Commission, Rose had every reason to believe that in the immediate future he would be offered the presidency of the new Peabody College for Teachers. Indeed, he was asked in early 1910, shortly after he had taken up his duties with the Sanitary Commission. The invitation to take charge of the Commission, then, came at a time when Rose not only had much unfinished business of his own in Nashville but also stood next in line to assume the highest position in the newly revitalized college to which he had devoted over twenty years of his life. With all this in mind, the question of why the Rockefeller people picked Rose seems less important – after all, they did want a highly respected and well-known Southern educator – than the question of why Rose accepted.[42]

Stiles left no record of what he thought of the man chosen to manage the Commission. His relationship with Rose was always outwardly correct, but the two men never struck up a friendship that went beyond the requirements of their respective positions. Rose shared few, if any, of the zoologist's tastes or interests. Unlike the blustering, obstreperous scientific secretary, Rose was modest and self-effacing to a fault. Nothing about his physical appearance commanded attention. Slightly below average height and somewhat slight of build, Rose was clean-shaven with regular, unremarkable features. He dressed neatly and conservatively and wore pince-nez to strengthen eyes grown weak over a lifetime of scholarship. Those who knew him only slightly were impressed by the strength and the precision of his intellect. Felix Frankfurter, for example, wrote that "Rose has one of the best trained minds I have ever seen in a layman. His understanding of the problems of modern law amazed us all." After one of Rose's visits to England for the International Health Commission, Sir Arthur Salter wrote Fosdick, "Who is this man Rose you sent me? He has one of the best economic minds I have ever met." Fosdick himself, impressed with Rose, remembered that Rose took his personal motto from Hegel's thesis that "reason is the substance of the universe."[43]

Logical and self-disciplined, certainly, Rose was also known to those who worked closely with him for his gentle patience, his unfailing courtesy, and his administrative flexibility. But perhaps he stood out from his colleagues most noticeably for his deep-seated reluctance to stand out at all. Unlike many of the men with whom he worked, Rose seemed to take genuine satisfaction in anonymity. He rarely gave interviews and strove hard to keep his name out of the public eye. His secretary found him detached and impersonal with everyone around the office: "He never seemed to take any interest in the private affairs of the staff, although he was correct and friendly in his office relations."[44] She recalled that he often stayed behind in the office after everyone else had gone home so that he could read without interruption.

His tastes in literature ran toward contemporary British poetry and fiction, a predilection that in itself marked him off from the rest of his associates. Masefield, Pater, and Arnold Bennett were among the authors he read after hours in his office and discussed at length in letters to friends back in Tennessee. He even tried his own hand at composition (in French) from time to time, affecting the lush, narcissistic style of the European *fin de siècle* aesthetes. It may be that he wrote poetry to maintain his fluency in French, but it is more likely that he was giving vent to a submerged poetic sensibility, one that could not find expression in the daily course of events at the Commission. The secretary who found him aloof and impersonal and typed hundreds of his flat, business-like letters to field workers would not have known what to make of "Les silences chantent à moi," one of the several poems written out in longhand and found in his private files.[45]

If Rose kept his private life completely to himself, it was no doubt because he found no kindred spirits among the Baptist ministers and public health doctors of the Rockefeller Sanitary Commission, at least no one who shared his taste for literature. He did, however, hold one passion in common with Gates. Both men were avid fishermen. Rose, in fact, following in Stiles's footsteps, accidentally discovered a new species of trout in the California Sierras, and in a rare departure from his usual modesty, allowed it to be named for him (*Salmo Rosei*).[46]

Rose brought only a layman's knowledge of medicine to his job, but he came to Washington with some definite ideas on how the campaign against hookworm disease should be conducted. Through the winter months of 1910, he mapped out the plan of attack and selected and deployed his personnel, while bearing in mind both the nature of the enemy and the stipulations of the Rockefeller office.

He, Gates, and Stiles agreed that the battle had to be waged on three coordinated fronts. First, agents of the Commission had to define the geographical distribution of the disease and come up with a reasonably accurate estimate of the degree of infection in each territorial unit. After the completion of this preliminary stage, the immediate victims of the infection must be cured. And, finally, Rose's staff must first contain, then obliterate the sources of hookworm infestation, and guard against the possibility of its return.[47]

In order to wage this three-pronged assault, the Commission had to decide upon a basic unit of organization, a liaison between the administrative officers and the workers in the field. In the past, the General Education Board had found its goals more readily fulfilled when the unit of organization was an already well-established instituion. As Rose pointed out, "in the interest both of economy and of efficiency . . . the work should be done as far as possible through existing agencies."[48] The members of the Commission, with the Board's experience before them, settled on the oldest, most venerated political unit in the South—the state. Each Southern state possessed a network of established agencies that could be brought to bear on the hookworm menace within its borders. Each had a public health office—in most cases, small and ineffectual; each had a system of organized medicine, public printing facilities, and schools.

The question of rightful jurisdiction also supported the selection of the state as the administrative go-between. Again, it was Rose who perceived the nuances of power and authority inherent in this consideration: "The economic prosperity of the State, the lives and health of its people, and the education of its children are involved; if the infection is to be stamped out, the States in which it exists must assume the responsibility. An outside agency can be helpful only in so far as it aids the States in organizing and bringing into activity their own forces."[49] In a region whose history was marred with incidents issuing from real or imagined imbalances between state and suprastate sovereignty, outside agencies had to take great care in carrying out their work behind the scenes, through the recognized seats of authority.

The Sanitary Commission found most of the state public health agencies inadequate to meet the demands of a rigorous state-wide campaign of the type necessary to do battle with the hookworm. Only six of the twelve Southern states[50] had continuous public health institutions in existence for more than a decade prior to the creation of the Sanitary Commission. Most of these six dated from the 1880s, with the oldest, Tennessee's, going back only as far as 1877.[51]

Florida alone provided its board of health with a stable fund
based on the mill system of taxation. The other eleven relied exclusively on legislative appropriations, at best a precarious
dependency. The Arkansas State Department of Health, for example, was organized in 1881, but as late as December 1910, had
yet to receive a cent for public health purposes. Its board was not
active, nor did it maintain an office.[52]

The specified legal qualifications and methods of appointment
of the state public health officers also served to dramatize the in-
significance attached to the agencies. Florida asked that its
officials only be "discreet citizens," but custom had always made
one out of the three a physician. Kentucky stipulated that all
eight must be legally qualified regular health practictioners of the
state; however, "One member must be a homeopath, one an
osteopath, one eclectic and the others allopathic physicians."[53] In
Arkansas, Georgia, Mississippi, Texas, and Virginia, the power
of appointment to the state board of health rested in the hands of
the governor. Florida, Kentucky, and Louisiana gave their chief
executives the right to nominate candidates, but called for senate
confirmation of his nominees. Only Alabama, North Carolina, and
South Carolina permitted the state medical associations a voice
in the appointments. Board positions in the other nine states
were often nothing more than political sinecures, filled by politicians on a patronage basis without regard to the medical
qualifications of the appointee. If a board were to discharge its
duties effectively, it might easily step on the toes of influential
people, in carrying out a quarantine, for instance, or condemning
a crop. Clearly public health officers should be not only capable,
experienced men of science and medicine, but state officials pro-
tected from undue political interference as well.

Only four states – Florida, Virginia, Louisiana, and Texas – empowered their boards of health to make and promulgate a
sanitary code carrying the weight of law. The other eight were
basically impotent. They could advise, caution, or propose
measures to the legislature for adoption into law, but they were
not legally equipped, in themselves, to see that their recommendations were carried out.

Possibly a more glaring deficiency in the South's public health
system was the lack of organization on the county level. As the
Commission discovered: "One of the most striking features of
these States systems of public health is the inefficiency of the
county health service."[54] Louisiana, perhaps the only state to
escape this indictment, had a fairly well-coordinated network of
parish health boards, but the state public health structure there

was rendered less effective than it might have been by political manipulation. Each local board in Louisiana was given the power to establish regulations in the form of laws, but since the parish board came under the general supervision of the state board, it had to make its regulations conform to those of the higher agency and satisfy the whims of the people in Baton Rouge.

In most of the remaining states, the county health officer, where there was on at all, took on the countywide responsibilities as an adjunct to his private practice, for his salary as the local public health officer amounted to very little. The Sanitary Commission concluded that the most feasible way to stimulate and utilize local initiative was by concentrating on the improvement of state and county boards. It went on to emphasize that "there can be no effective health service in the county on any basis until there is in the county a capable health officer devoting his whole time to the service . . . The work is not going to be done until the man is paid an adequate salary for his services."[55]

If the Commission found the structure of public health institutions in the South lacking, it soon discovered the region's attitude toward work of this kind needed reorientation as well. Southerners had come to regard their public health services as relief-bringing agencies, arriving on the scene of an epidemic or a natural disaster to repair the damages and ameliorate the suffering. For wherever Southern land touched the sea – along the marshy lowlands of the South Atlantic or throughout the bayou backcountry of the Gulf Coast – hurricanes, malaria, and yellow fever wreaked periodic havoc on the coastal inhabitants. Travelers to the region had long wondered how people could live under such conditions. Frederick Law Olmsted, one of its better-known visitors, noted in the 1850s: "The unacclimated whites on the sea coast and on the river and bayou banks of the low country, between which and the sea coast there is much inter-communication, suffer greatly from certain epidemic pestilences."[56] David F. Houston, of the Commission's board of directors, remarked to Page over dinner on the night of Rockefeller's announcement that most of the country of the lowland South was unfit for white residence. So much a part of life in the South were these seasonal calamities that native Southerners accepted them as just another price paid for living in the region. The several state public health agencies were set up not in an attempt to prevent calamities but to mitigate the ensuing misery and destruction. After the turn of the century, when it became known that epidemics of malaria and yellow fever could be checked before they started, public health officers found their hands tied through lack of funds and legal authority. Popular attitudes still viewed public health services as special, remedial organizations—regional Red Crosses—with only *post hoc* powers.[57]

Such was the state of public health work in the South when the Commission set out to conquer the hookworm. Small, understaffed, without sufficient funds or public support to do their jobs correctly, the struggling public health bureaus of the Southern states were in need of a stimulus of some sort. Rose and Gates knew this. Despit the fact that the General Education Board had already worked out an elaborate network of contacts and built up a sizable fund of goodwill among Southern school systems, and despite the fact that Rose and over half the members of the board of directors were widely known educators, the Sanitary Commission decided from the first to provide the needed boost to the state boards of health by carrying out its work through them.[58]

# 6

# Making the
# Idea Fashionable

Apart from his personal physician in Nashville, very few doctors in the South had heard of Wickliffe Rose in early January 1910. One of his first actions as the new administrative secretary of the Rockefeller Sanitary Commission, therefore, was to invite several hundred prominent physicians and state public health officials from the twelve Southern states to attend a conference in Atlanta. The meeting, it was hoped, would serve a twofold introductory purpose: he and they would get a chance to meet and size each other up, and they would have an opportunity to learn firsthand what the Commission proposed to do. Rose was extremely pleased to see some five hundred people representing eighteen states turn up in Atlanta on such short notice for the opening session of the conference on January 18, 1910. He himself arrived straight from the January 15 meeting of the Commission's board of directors in New York, at which he had been officially confirmed in his new position.[1]

Rose found the mood of the gathering "serious, hopeful, and aggressive" and came away with the feeling that the Commission had been well launched. Most of those in attendance had been previously unaware of the dimensions of the menace posed by hookworm disease to the citizens of their respective states. One delegation, however, returned home somewhat disappointed that they had not heard anything new; the contingent of doctors from Florida left the Atlanta conference convinced that they knew more than the Rockefeller agents about the practical aspects of conducting an anti-hookworm campaign. The eleven other Southern states represented at the conference all got around sooner or later to requesting the assistance of the Commission, but Florida remained aloof for the very good reason that it did not need any help. The Florida State Board of Health had recently embarked on a vigorous fight against hookworm disease on its own initiative with funds set aside from state taxes, and rather than soliciting the cooperation of the Rockefeller Sanitary Commission in their work, the Floridians generously and somewhat proudly invited Rose and his fledgling state directors to visit Florida for some on-the-job training.[2]

In 1909 the Florida State Board of Health had found itself suffering from an embarrassment of riches. The state public health officer, Dr. Joseph Y. Porter, had sequestered a substantial reserve from his past few budgets against the day when Florida would be hit with another yellow fever epidemic. In the meantime, the one-half mill per tax dollar allocated for public health work in the state had generated $75,000 in 1909 alone. By comparison, the average amount appropriated by the eleven other Southern state legislatures in the same year was a relatively meager $17,000. Other branches of the Florida state government had begun to eye Porter's burgeoning reserves with envy. It was shortly after a small raid by the bureau in charge of pensions for Civil War veterans that Porter sanctioned the creation of a program to combat hookworm disease.[3]

Thanks to the information flowing from Porter's office, Florida physicians had been aware of the parasite in their midst for about six years before the budget surplus crisis. Dr. Hiram Byrd, Porter's assistant, had begun to collect data on hookworm from doctors in the Tampa area shortly after the publication of Stiles's *Report upon the Prevalence and Geographic Distribution of Hookworm Disease in the United States* (1902). At the same time, Byrd initiated a survey to uncover the extent of hookworm disease in Florida. For the next five years, the board of health kept physicians and interested laymen on its mailing lists abreast of new developments in the detection and treatment of hookworm disease. In December 1908, it began a program in the public schools in cooperation with the Florida State Teachers' Association. Byrd estimated that of the 285,000 children of school age in Florida, over 200,000 lived in conditions that virtually guaranteed their exposure to hookworm disease. Six months after the public school program began, Porter released funds to implement a scheme designed to reimburse general practitioners from treating indigent hookworm victims. Once a diagnosis had been confirmed in a state laboratory and after the record of the case had been filed with the state board, a payment of three dollars was authorized as a matter of course. Such a plan would not threaten, but would in fact bolster, a physician's private practice. Two weeks before Rockefeller's letter to the Sanitary Commission's board of directors, Porter hired two full-time doctors to reinforce the voluntary aspects of his coordinated attack on hookworm disease. Doctors E. W. Diggett and C. T. Young traveled from county to county, visiting in schools, churches, and private homes, surveying the extent of infection in each locality, and encouraging people to seek treatment from a local doctor. By the time of Rose's Atlanta conference, the Florida State Board of Health employed over forty people, maintained three laboratories in three different cities, and regularly mailed issues of its own publication, *Florida Health Notes,* to public school teachers and the approximately one thousand physicians across the state. Porter and Byrd were just beginning to get a clear sense of what they were up against when Rose invited them to Atlanta. They were pleased to see the battle joined on other fronts but remained skeptical that $1 million would go very far if spread over eleven states. Still, they encouraged Rose and his state directors to visit Florida and study their methods. Porter also agreed to send quarterly reports to Rose's office for inclusion in the Sanitary Commission's annual report.[4]

Shortly after his trip to Florida, Rose got another opportunity to evaluate in person a different program already in place. Stiles certainly knew who Bailey Ashford was and had heard of his work in Puerto Rico, but it does not appear that he ever mentioned it to his associates at the Rockefeller Sanitary Commission. Shortly after Rose's appointment, however, Lyman Abbott, editor-in-chief of *The Outlook,* wrote a letter to Welch detailing at length the story of Ashford's ten-year campaign against hookworm disease on the island. Welch forwarded the letter to Gates, who in turn passed it along to Rose. In February 1910, while Rose was back in Nashville seeing to the arrangements for his family's removal to Washington, his assistant, A. P. Bourland, met with President Taft and Secretary of War J. M. Dickinson to discuss the work of the Rockefeller Sanitary Commission vis-à-vis Ashford's Anemia Commission of Puerto Rico. Bourland encouraged Rose to visit Ashford and reported that the Secretary of War was willing to provide him with a letter of introduction to the governor of Puerto Rico. The only sour note struck during Bourland's meeting with Taft and Dickinson concerned the ever-controversial Stiles. The administration, in Bourland's opinion, believed that Ashford had been robbed of his rightful due as the discover of hookworm disease in North America. Bourland concluded that, "As matters are now we will

not get much if any cooperation from the government outside of
Dr. S's sphere of influence whereas we need it largely." He urged
Rose to go to Puerto Rico as soon as possible and to give serious
thought to the possibility of extending the work of the Commission in that direction. "By taking up the Puerto Rico work we will
get cooperation and all the benefits of Ashford's work."[5]

Rose sailed for Puerto Rico on May 29, 1910, after his tour of
Florida. He spent three weeks on the island in the company of
Ashford and the men of the Puerto Rico Commission visiting
clinics and absorbing the details of their well-established program. Ashford also furnished him with a list of names and addresses of people – most of whom he knew personally – who were
treating or studying hookworm disease overseas, in Oxford, London, Liège, Brussels, Padua, Germany, Madrid, and Cairo. Rose
came away from his tour thoroughly impressed and leaning
toward an extension of the Sanitary Commission's work into
Puerto Rico. He could not authorize such a move on his own initiative, but he did discuss it freely with both Ashford and the
governor of the island. According to Rose, Governor George Colton "seemed very desirous that something, however small, might
be done by way of recognition of what had already been done and
of the importance of making larger contributions to this service.
It was his judgment that the spirit of cooperation thus manifested would be of more value than any financial assistance involved."[6] Both Colton and Ashford made it clear to Rose that
they would not be averse to the idea of financial assistance as
well. Back in Washington, Rose wrote Ashford: "My whole experience in Porto Rico grows upon me as the days go by ... To
you I owe the very unusual opportunity which I had to see Porto
Rico, its people and its problems."[7]

What had Rose seen and learned in Puerto Rico? Ashford had
returned to the island in 1902 after a tour of duty in New York
and, in association with Dr. W. W. King of the Marine Hospital
Service, had immediately set aside two wards in the Ponce
hospital for hookworm sufferers. He and King published a report,
based on one hundred cases arising from their work on the wards,
which caused a slight stir on the island. Ashford followed this up
with an address before the Medical Association of Puerto Rico in
December of the same year. In 1903, the governor of the island,
William H. Hunt, allocated $5,000 for hookworm work, to be
directed by a commission made up of Ashford, King, and a native
Puerto Rican physician, Pedro Gutiérrez Igaravídez. On March 6,
1904, the Anemia Commission in Puerto Rico opened a tent

hospital in Bayamon with equipment on loan from the Army Medical Corps. In the course of the next year, the hospital was taken to several other towns and cities and treated a total of 5,490 persons, of whom 2,244 were reported cured, 377 partially cured, and 1,727 improved; 27 people died in the hospital. Because of a tight budget, the members of the Anemia Commission could only admit the most serious hookworm disease sufferers for treatment in the hospital. The rest were taken on an out-patient basis. In 1905 the governor trebled the appropriation to $15,000. The number of persons treated in that year accordingly increased threefold to 18,865. Ashford was ordered to resume his regular duties with the Army in 1906, and King was sent back to the quarantine service, but a new commission made up entirely of Puerto Ricans under the direction of Gutiérrez continued the work. By the time of Rose's visit, a quarter of a million patients had been treated by the Anemia Commission in the six years since its creation, but there still remained a larger number of hookworm victims on the island who had not been reached.[8]

The War Department, at Ashford's and Colton's request, was in the process of asking Congress to take over and increase the annual appropriations so that the work could be continued and expanded. Ashford and Gutiérrez felt that the mobile field hospitals and clinics served admirably as emergency treatment centers and as terminals for the distribution of information, but that reinfection threatened to undo a portion of their work unless a much larger effort was mounted to improve the sanitary conditions of the *jibaros'* villages and farms. In 1902 Ashford had estimated that fully 30 percent of all deaths in Puerto Rico were attributable in varying degrees to hookworm disease, either directly or subtly as the contributing agent, by weakening the victim and leaving him more vulnerable to other illnesses which, but for the presence of hookworms in large numbers, might not be fatal. He could point with pride eight years later to the statistics which indicated that the death rate from hookworm disease had been cut in half, or in some coffee districts by more than half, since the Anemia Commission went into business. But he warned that without greatly increased funding sufficient to launch a large-scale sanitation improvement program, hookworm disease would reassert its control over the poorer inhabitants of the island just as surely and just as swiftly as the Puerto Rican jungle reclaimed an abandoned coffee plantation. What funds the Anemia Commission could normally expect were now in danger of being diverted to meet an unexpected and even more deadly intruder. "The worst of the present situation," Ashford wrote, "is that the resources of the island are being strained tremendously to meet the necessities of general sanitation and, lately, a special emergency in the shape of bubonic plague, a few cases of which have appeared for the first time in the history of the Island, has suddenly presented itself with all of the heavy expense it entails."[9] So much had been accomplished, yet in early 1910 it appeared to Ashford that much of it might be lost. Small wonder that the emissary of the Rockefeller philanthropies found the red carpet out for his arrival. After his tour of Ashford's beleaguered project, Rose thanked his host for "the unbounded courtesies you extended to me." Ashford needed all the help he could get.

Rose certainly admired what Ashford had accomplished in Puerto Rico, and he seems to have struck up an immediate friendship with Ashford as well. "It was a great joy to know you personally," he wrote, "and to meet your family. When you come to Washington I hope to have you in my own home."[10] At Rose's insistence, Ashford did come to the United States in late 1910, and with funds furnished by the Rockefeller Sanitary Commission, gave a well-publicized series of lectures in the Southern states to discuss his work in Puerto Rico. Rose sent him up to New York to meet Page and to supply background material for an article on the hookworm to appear in *World's Work*. Stiles could just as easily have done both, but Rose was coming to rely on him for as little as possible in the area of public relations.[11]

When he wrote the job description for the scientific secretary, Gates had tried to reduce the number of ways in which Stiles could injure the reputation or tarnish the image of the Sanitary Commission, but the zoologist found the means to do both despite the limitations of his office. Rose came quickly to learn that Stiles could still anger people in the name of the Commission. His very reputation as the "discoverer" of hookworm disease irritated the Secretary of War, who felt that Ashford could lay better claim to that distinction. Gates had warned Rose that Stiles's membership on the board of directors might draw the wrath of the anti-child-labor forces and had arranged it so that Stiles himself, in a stylized act of public contrition, introduced the resolution at the January 15, 1910, annual meeting stating that the question of child labor was one with which the Commission would not be concerned. Even so, Rose soon discovered that Stiles had not mended his ways, and worse still, that he, Rose, was now being asked, sometimes by old friends, to account for Stiles's behavior. Edgar Gardner Murphy, head of the National

Child Labor Committee, was one such old friend. It had been he who first introduced Rose to the Southern Education Board and nominated him to be its Executive Secretary. Murphy learned of a speech that Stiles had given in Boston in late January 1910, in which the child-labor issue had been raised once again. Shortly afterwards, Murphy was able to confront Stiles in person at a meeting of the Union League Club in New York where Page had been asked to speak. Stiles's personal views were bad enough, Murphy believed, but when he expressed them as the official representative of the Rockefeller Sanitary Commission they became intolerable. In a letter to Rose, he neatly summarized the fears of all anti-child-labor activists:

Now, as to Dr. Stiles. My questions the other other evening were asked with too much asperity – an asperity they would have lacked had I known his remarks on the child labor question (repeatedly published for nearly two years) had occasioned any definite correction from his associates on the hook-worm commission. Long after the members of the Commission were called together for organization in New York, he continued these remarks – until their culmination in his recent speech in Boston. Through all this period he has been in close contact with Mr. Gates and with other representatives of the Commission and – as he has had the center of the stage – it was altogether natural for some of us to fear that the great power of the Rockefeller endowments (at least indirectly) might be turned against us in the struggle for decent factory legislation in the South. As the "discoverer" of hook-worm, Dr. Stiles will always command great popular interest and influence; men like Dr. Alderman, Dr. Houston, Dr. Page, and yourself would not oppose the legislative protection of children in industry; but it will be a long time before Dr. Stiles will cease (popularly) to be the real representative of the hook-worm propaganda. This impression will gradually be corrected; outsiders (like myself) who at least *try* to be men of discrimination will in due time learn the truth. But we have all done a good deal of "waiting"; and misunderstanding, and even "asperities" (in view of certain wholly personal criticisms that some of us have had to endure) have not been unnatural.[12]

Part of Stiles's problem stemmed from his habit of being blunt on purpose in the hope of arousing his listeners from their apathy, a strategy in which he persisted long after it became clear that the shocks he administered often produced an undesirable effect. At an address before the second annual Child Conference for Research and Welfare, meeting in Worcester, Massachusetts, in late June and early July 1910, Stiles studiously avoided any mention of the child-labor issue, but his opening remarks still managed to antagonize his audience. "In our national conceit," he stated, "we Americans imagine that we lead the world in almost any field that can be mentioned. After an experience of seven years residence and travel among other civilized nationalities . . . I am unable to escape the conclusion that, taken as a nation, we Americans are dirtier than any of the other civilized nations with which I have come into close contact."[13] No doubt the sanitary habits of many Americans in 1910 would not have stood close scrutiny, but the gentlemen in starched collars who listened to Stiles's address did not take lightly his charge that they were jingoistic, self-deluded, and filthy.

Reports from other quarters left little doubt in Rose's mind that Stiles's abrasiveness was alienating people outside the circle of anti-child-labor activists as well. A Richmond public health official, later active in the hookworm work, wrote that although he himself had not been present when Stiles read a paper before the Conference of State and Territorial Boards of Health in Washington, he "had been told by three parties who were present that the paper was of a sensational nature and implied threats against the South if the hookworm was not promptly eradicated . . . Such an attitude and statements can seriously interfere and handicap the work now attempted by your Commission and the Boards of Health." Rose's worried correspondent concluded that "the people will listen to quiet reasoning and will take necessary measures recommended by local physicians, but should an outsider attempt by sensational statements and threats to force the people to adopt preventive measures, the whole question will be disparaged and attempts at improvement be resisted."[14]

Even Stiles's heavy-handed attempts at humor upset people. A field worker in North Carolina remembered that Stiles would often go before county boards to urge them to hire full-time health officers. Stiles would then add: "And he need not be a relative of the County Health Commissioner." The field worker recognized, as Stiles apparently did not, that "since there was usually a relative or two of the Commissioner on the Board, this seldom went over very well."[15]

Stiles remained a thorn of sorts in Rose's side even after he transferred to the Public Health Service hospital in Wilmington, North Carolina, midway through the Commission's campaign. One of the circulars bearing his signature accused the mothers of Wilmington, through their failure to grasp the rudiments of sanitation, of literally feeding their children human excrement.[16]

If Stiles could be muzzled, his critics might yet become strong supporters of the Commission. Murphy had said as much. The task of winning over the large and highly vocal minority of Southerners who despised the very idea of the Commission would not be as simple. Rose had been in Nashville when the announcement of the new Rockefeller benefaction hit the newspapers, and he had noted the mixed sentiments with which it was greeted. Shortly after he accepted the job of administrative secretary, he told Gates of his fear that the Commission might run into serious opposition in the South. A year later, in his first annual report, he recalled that "The announcement that hookworm is prevalent in the States was not taken seriously. Many people resented the suggestion of their being infected and refused to be examined and treated."[17] Four years later, in referring to the reaction of the Southern press at the outset of the campaign, Rose wrote: "Some of them [Southern newspapers in late 1909 and early 1910] denounced the assertion that such a disease existed at all. Many were particularly bitter in disclaiming its existence in the South."[18] Both of these matter-of-fact statements fail to convey the intensity of the furor that raged throughout the region's newspapers, its pulpits, and on the floors of its legislative halls following the announcement of the Commission's formation. Whereas before, when Stiles revealed his discovery in 1902, press reaction had been benignly whimsical, now a large number of Southern editors and public men were indignant.

"Where was this hookworm or lazy disease, when it took five Yankee soldiers to whip one Southerner?" asked the *Macon* (Georgia) *Telegraph*.[19] B. E. Washburn, a sanitary investigator in North Carolina, recalled one ingenious allegation: "One theory advanced was that Mr. Rockefeller was preparing to go into the shoe business and had financed the hookworm campaign as a preliminary move to scare the people of the South into wearing shoes at all times and not in the winter season alone."[20] An article in the *Arkansas Democrat* reporting on the debate in the state legislature on a public health bill told of a certain Mr. Gray who rose on the floor of the legislature to denounce the bill, claiming that "the doctors' trust had conspired with the leather trust, several years ago, and invented the great bugaboo of the hookworm so that poor people had to wear more shoes."[21] Richard Hathaway Edmonds' influential New South journal, the *Manufacturers' Record*, saw the hookworm announcement as the latest tactic in a Northern conspiracy to rob the South of business: "At the turn of the century the beginning was made with the agitation, principally false, about 'child labor' in Southern mills ... Dovetailed with this was the 'educational' movement picturing as an excuse for itself the South as a region of ignorance and poverty, and dovetailing with both was the 'hookworm' propaganda, picturing the South as a place of ill-health and disease."[22] If Stiles saw this editorial, he must have been grimly amused to see himself included in the same conspiracy with the anti-child-labor people. The *Manufacturers' Record* went on to ask: "With nearly every paper in the country heralding the South as the peculiar home of the 'hookworm,' and full of its dangers to life, how many settlers can turn from other regions to this section?"[23] The *Charlote News*, less analytical than the *Manufacturers' Record*, simply called the Commission a "body of fanatics."[24]

Josephus Daniels of the *Raleigh News and Observer* felt that the Rockefeller Sanitary Commission was just another manifestation of the Country Life Commission he had decried only a year earlier. He remembered Stiles from the Roosevelt Commission's public hearing in Raleigh in November 1908, and he had noted with disgust that the *Report of the Commission On Country Life*, submitted to the President in January 1909 and passed on by him to the Congress, had repeated Stiles's contentions verbatim, without editorial caution. Hookworm disease, that earlier Commission had concluded, was a major detrimental factor in the South's farm labor situation. Congress, in Daniels' view, had very wisely buried the *Report* without fanfare, and President Taft showed little inclination to disinter it. Now, a disreputable Northern robber baron with a penchant for meddling had taken it upon himself to do what the government had chosen not to. Daniels editorialized: "Many of us in the South are getting tired of being exploited by advertisements that exaggerate conditions. They are most harmful. As to hookworm, this paper has accepted the statement of the widespread prevalence of that disease with many grains of allowance. Let us not canonize Standard Oil Rockefeller by putting laurels on his head because he seeks to buy the appreciation of the people whom he has been robbing for a quarter of a century."[25]

The columnist Irving Cobb raised the spectre of the carpetbagger when he wondered whether Southerners wanted hookworm "dispossessed from their midst by a rank outsider from the North."[26] Perhaps the most powerful critic of the Sanitary Commission was the Social Gospel Methodist Bishop of Georgia, Warren A. Candler, author of the widely read *Great Revivals and the Great Republic* and brother of the founder and guiding light of the Coca-Cola company. Candler, who saw the Commission as a Trojan Horse designed to take over Southern education, joined the rising chorus of denunciations by predicting, "The Southern people will not be taken in by Mr. Rockefeller's vermifuge fund and hookworm commission."[27] Two years later, even after he had come to accept the presence of hookworm disease among his parishioners and to admire the efforts of Georgia's doctors to combat it, Candler still resented Rockefeller's hand in the undertaking. When invited by Dr. A. M. Wood, a Georgia field worker in the hookworm campaign, to visit a dispensary in the little town of Sparks, Candler declined, saying, "But I know what you are doing, and that it is a most excellent work, but let us do these things ourselves and give Mr. Rockefeller back his money."[28]

Although expressed in a number of imaginative ways, the hostile reaction to the creation of the Rockefeller Sanitary Commission came down to one fundamental attitude: We don't believe there is such a thing as widespread hookworm infection in the South; the whole business is just another confounded Yankee trick to weaken and to ridicule the South; but even if hookworm did exist here, we would certainly prefer to do something about it ourselves rather than to have John D. Rockefeller do it for us.

Gates tended to play down the virulence and underestimate the potential impact of opposition to the Commission. He told Rose that both the Southern Education Board and the General Education Board had encountered a small amount of hostility from certain quarters when they were first getting under way, but he labeled it "sporadic . . . and feeble." He warned Rose to expect opposition from Candler, "who opposed everything in the way of assistance to the South from every source." He also thought that "there are one or two fire-eating papers which agree with him." But the preponderance of Southern "organs of opinion" welcomed the Commission with "gratitude and approval" in a manner that has been "practically universal and overwhelming."[29] Gates also told Rose of the scrapbook of newspaper clippings he had started after the announcement of the Commission's creation.

Candler and Daniels did not speak for most Southerners. Gates overlooked, however, the damage that a few important men could inflict on the Commission. Candler probably influenced Georgia's Senator Hoke Smith to oppose and eventually defeat the bill in the United States Senate to charter the Rockefeller Foundation. James K. Vardaman of Mississippi, although he soon came to support the Commission enthusiastically, initially published Candler's attack, with approving comments of his own, in his newspaper. Vardaman's stature in Mississippi alone would seem to indicate that opposition to the Commission came from more than Candler and "one or two fire-eating newspapers." In Texas, Governor Thomas M. Campbell blocked all Commission activities for as long as he held office.[30]

Dr. Olin West, state director of the hookworm campaign in Tennessee, summarized what he thought to be the underlying causes of the antagonism to the Sanitary Commission in his state, but he might as well have been speaking of the whole South. Rockefeller's association with the work, in his opinion, guaranteed a certain amount of vociferous opposition. Candler's "very scathing" article, "in which . . . he denounces the Commission and everyone connected therewith, denying the prevalence of Hookworm Disease and ridiculing the statements of authorities concerning the effects produced by it, holding up to scorn the germ theory, and otherwise disporting himself in print," had also been undeniably damaging, in West's view. He reserved his last indictment for what he saw as exaggerated newspaper and magazine articles, "especially those appearing in Northern periodicals."[31]

West's last point was well taken. Newspapers in the rest of the country may have done as much to kindle a hostile reaction in the Southern press as did the actual creation of the Commission. Rather than treat the campaign for what it was, several of them lapsed into their old satirical attitude. Walt Mason, a syndicated pundit with a wide national following, assumed a jeering posture in one of his columns:

He was a mournful looking wreck, with yellow face and scrawny neck, and weary eyes that looked as though they had monopoly of woe. Too tired to get his labors done, all day he loitered in the sun, and filled the air with yawns and moans, while people called him Lazybones. One day the doctor came, and said: "Brace up, my friend! Hold up your head! The hookworm deadly as an asp, has got you in its loathesome grasp! But I will break the hookworm loose, and cook its everlasting goose! Swing wide your mouth, and do not cringe —" and then he took his big syringe, and shot about a quart of dope, that tasted like a bar of soap, adown the patient's yawning throat — "I guess I got that hookworm's goat!" One gasping breath the patient drew, and bit a lightning rod in two, and vaulted o'er his cottage roof: and then, on nimble, joyous hoof he sped across the wind-swept plain, and burned a school and robbed a train. The doctor watched his patient streak across the landscape sere and bleak, and said "it makes my bosom warm. What wonders Science can perform."[32]

It is not difficult to see why an already sensitive South would recoil in the face of such mockery.

At least as galling to proud Southerners was the abundant pity proffered by right-thinking progressive Northerners. Years after the work of the Sanitary Commission was done, E. E. Cummings ridiculed the sense of fuzzy sympathy that he remembered from his Massachusetts boyhood. Safely shod and far north of the hookworm belt in any event, the youthful Cummings had exercised his precocious talents for the pleasure of his teachers at the Cambridge High and Latin School—and the other Cambridge ladies he later came to detest—by writing poems about the hookworm campaign in which he implored "healthy Christians to assist poor-whites afflicted with The Curse of The Worm (short for hookworm)."[33] By contrast, there was nothing sympathetic in the reaction of that transplanted Northerner, Mark Twain, to the hookworm controversy. Bitter and sardonic towards the end of his life, Twain found ample material in the whole episode to fuel his savage wit. In a lengthy passage in the early pages of *Letters from the Earth*, he recounted the story of Dr. Stiles and the Rockefeller gift. His object was to mount a double-barreled attack upon God, for creating hookworms in the first place and then for taking credit for helping to eradicate them.[34]

Walter Hines Page was predictably extolling the merits of the Commission in *World's Work* on every possible occasion. Armed with an endless supply of superlatives, he paraded article after article through the pages of his magazine, all as guilty of exaggerating the value of the Commission's work as any of the Southern "fire-eating" papers were of underestimating it. He genuinely believed that in unmasking the hookworm Stiles had isolated the South's curse, the single black thread tracing its way through the region's history and dooming it to poverty, defeat, and ignorance. "The discovery . . . of hookworm disease in the United States is the most helpful event in the history of the Southern states . . . The hookworm has probably played a larger part in our Southern history than slavery or wars or any political dogma or economic creed."[35] Slave owners and the society that included them might still be condemned by some for moral turpitude, but they could no longer be accused of stupidity. It had not been their willful and conscious persistence in a ruinous practice that had brought the house down upon their heads or doomed their children to penury. An unrecognized curse of truly Biblical proportions had done the job. Now that the Sanitary Commission was hard at work, Page foresaw the curtain going up on a new, prosperous era in the life of the nation, with his own region restored to its rightful place in the sun as the dreadful scourge of hookworm was driven from the land. "Every man who knows the people of the Southern states sees in the results of this work a new epoch in their history and, because of its sanitary suggestiveness, a new epoch in our national history . . . Now for the first time, the main cause of their long backwardness is explained and it is a removable cause."[36]

The *Macon Telegraph*, the same paper that had counted the number of Yankees it took to subdue one Confederate, would have none of Page's *uncinaria fecit* theory of history: "The prospect of a reconstruction of history and theology on a hookworm basis is scarcely inviting, but there is left us at least the consolation that some new discovery will in good time dethrone the little intestinal parasite, or relegate it to its proper and relatively unimportant place, and at the same time send many of the fine-spun theories of traveling enthusiasts to the dump heap."[37] Other well-known journalists besides Page—among them Lyman Abbott and Ray Stannard Baker—published articles on the campaign in magazines with national circulations such as *The Outlook* and the *American Magazine*. Rose contended that Page's articles always brought more inquiries to his office than any of the rest.[38]

While the journalists were locked in their private but fascinating aerial combat, Rose was methodically marshaling his troops for the war in the trenches. In the year 1910, nine states invited the support of the Commission in inaugurating a campaign against hookworm disease. Work first began in Virginia on February 7. Eight other Southern states were quick to follow the lead. North Carolina (March 12), Georgia (April 20), South Carolina (May 1), Tennessee (May 10), Arkansas (May 10), Mississippi (June 1), Alabama (October 1), and Louisiana (November 1), were all engaged in the work, with the Commission's aid, by the year's end.[39]

For each of the states enlisted in the work, a director of sanitation was appointed. To fill this position, the Sanitary Commission, in close conjunction with the chairman of the state board of health, always selected a physician already with, or soon to become a member of, the state department of health. The advantages of this rule of thumb were twofold and obvious: not only was the man chosen a resident of the state and a member of its medical establishment, but he was also well acquainted with the peculiar workings and specific limitations of his state's board of health. The state director (the title varied from state to state in an attempt to conform to each state's particular custom) was ultimately responsible for the efficiency of the work in his jurisdiction. He reported quarterly to his state board of health and, through the state board, to the Commission. Each director was also regularly in touch with Rose directly. His formal reports were circulated among the other state directors in order to keep them all abreast of innovations as well as of progress in the rest of the states. These quarterly reports engendered a kind of rivalry that was not always entirely friendly.

Rose had a clear idea from the outset of the kind of person he wanted to fill the state director's post. "I should like a young man who has unusual energy, who has had large clinical experience and is thoroughly familiar with all diseases that would be involved in the question of Public Health. He ought to have administrative powers. He will have to be at the head of an army of workers over the whole state and he should be a forceful personality, a man of thorough scientific temper; one who would command the respect of his profession and of the public at large."[40] Despite the fact that no work could begin in a state until a director had been chosen, Rose moved very methodically, almost slowly, through the interviewing and selection process. In the early months of 1910, he visited the states that had asked for the Commission's assistance, conferred with the men in charge of the state boards of health, and met with the various candidates. His deliberate pace brought long-lasting and satisfactory results. Of the nine state directors selected in 1910, seven remained at their jobs for the duration of the Commission's five-year life. One (Morgan Smith in Arkansas) quit to become the dean of his state's medical college; the other (John A. Ferrell of North Carolina) moved up to become Rose's assistant at the Commission's headquarters. Two of the original nine eventually achieved prominence in the public health field in their own right — Ferrell again, with the Rockefeller Foundation, and Allen W. Freeman of Virginia as a professor at the Johns Hopkins School of Public Health. Olin West of Tennessee later became the president of the American Medical Association. When Kentucky took up the work in 1911, Rose chose as his state director Arthur T. McCormack, son of Joseph N. McCormack, "the most influential leader of the profession in the Progressive Era" (in the opinion of an historian of the American Medical Association) on the strength of his eleven-year campaign to organize physicians on behalf of the AMA. For a man with no experience in medical or public health matters, Rose came remarkably close to finding a group of young doctors who met his exacting requirements.[41]

Each director of sanitation was equipped with a corps of inspectors, microscopists, and laboratory technicians. People staffing these positions were hired at the state level and paid by the Commission, through the state boards of health, on a full-time basis, primarily for work either in the field or in the state's public health laboratories. The director himself chose his staff, but his nominees for the positions of sanitary inspectors had to be approved by both his state health bureau and the Commission. All licensed physicians, the sanitary inspectors (or field workers) constituted the lifeblood of the campaign. They were the Commission's shock troops, trained and equipped to handle most aspects of its work. In his first annual report, Rose said of these sanitary inspectors:

They are the long arms with which the State director reaches out over the State to determine the geographic distribution and degree of infection; to determine the sanitary conditions responsible for the presence and spread of the disease; to enlist the cooperation of the physicians in curing the sufferers; to provide the treatment for the indigent; to inspect the schools; to instruct the teachers; enlist the press; and, by lectures, demonstrations, and personal conferences, teach the people the importance of getting all infected persons cured, and how to prevent the spread of disease by putting a stop to soil pollution.[42]

Clearly, the quality of the work done in any one state was largely contingent on the ability and energy of its force of sanitary inspectors. The only aspect of the Commission's activities in which they did not figure directly was the purely administrative. They reported regularly to the state director of sanitation and periodically submitted comprehensive reports on their progress. By the end of 1910, twenty-nine doctors in eight Southern states were on the rolls of the Sanitary Commission as inspectors.[43]

They were all young men in their twenties or early thirties, and all were Southerners who had been educated close to home. That they were committed to the people of their region is perhaps best illustrated by the remarkable fact that almost all who were alive in 1939 (and responded to a Rockefeller Foundation survey) were still practicing in the South. At first, Rose allowed several established physicians to become sanitary inspectors without giving up their private practices. The very first field worker, in fact, was a popular country doctor from the Northern Neck of Virginia. Rose quickly came to doubt, however, the wisdom of permitting the field workers to keep their practices. He continued to sanction the hiring of established physicians but only on condition that they be willing to devote all their time to the work of the Commission. The state director of North Carolina experimented with the idea of hiring traveling salesmen from the larger, more reputable drug houses to serve as his field workers when their other duties permitted. Rose strongly discouraged this practice on the grounds that whatever advantages such salesmen might bring to the campaign in "their skill in knowing and handling doctors in their practice and business relations" would be outweighed by the disadvantages of a staff of field workers with divided, even if compatible, loyalties. If most of the field workers were hired right out of medical school, this was because few established doctors were willing to give up their incomes from private practice for the $1,200-a-year starting salay offered by the Commission. Even so, Rose realized that "where you can find a reasonable young physician practicing in the country, commanding the respect of the people and already interested in hookworm disease, he seems to make an ideal field worker."[44] Rose was eager to see the work under way in each state as soon as possible but not at the risk of hiring people hastily. He wrote the director of the Alabama State Board of Health that although "the ultimate purpose is to have one man for each district," for the time being "it would not be wise to get all of these at work at once. It has been found in other states to be better to bring the men into the service somewhat gradually."[45] Younger men were less likely to be burdened with families and local responsibilities and would presumably be more mobile and more flexible. Young men, in Gates's opinion at least, were less likely to be bunglers, since they had received their medical training after the turn of the century.[46]

In addition to providing his salary and traveling expenses, the Commission furnished each sanitary inspector with a kit of working tools. This included a collapsible microscope, designed by Bausch and Lomb to fit in a saddlebag, a supply of medicine, popular literature for distribution among the curious, photographs and charts to illustrate day-time lectures, and a lantern with slides for use in the evening. Most of the men carried cameras, which they provided themselves, for making their own before-and-after photographs. They found, not surprisingly, that the impact of these visual aids increased noticeably when the subjects in the pictures were the friends and neighbors of the people in the audience.[47]

To round out each state director's staff of people engaged in the hookworm work, the Commission provided funds to improve a state laboratory or in some cases to assist in the construction of one, and to hire and train microscopists. Once the work was well under way in a state, microscopists were needed both in the field with the sanitary inspectors and back in the state laboratory.

Otherwise, the much more expensive field workers would have to spend time in analyzing samples that could be better spent drumming up business. The turnover in microscopists was rapid chiefly because they received low salaries – $40 a month to start with an incremental raises up to a ceiling of $50. Once they gained experience, the Commission-trained microscopists usually received offers for better-paying jobs outside the hookworm campaign. Since there does not seem to have been a dearth of applicants for the microscopists' positions, Rose could take twofold satisfaction in the knowledge that he was keeping expenses down while at the same time increasing each state's pool of trained and experienced technicians. Kentucky, which took up the hookworm work in 1911, introduced a cost-saving idea that was soon adopted in several other states. Originally, the Kentucky state director, Arthur T. McCormack, employed medical students on vacation to man the microscopes in the state laboratory. At the suggestion of the state bacteriologist who was in charge of the laboratory, Dr. Lillian Smith, he began to hire women to replace the students as they returned to school. He wrote that the women "do better work, do it faster, and are more satisfactory in every way."[48] One way in which the penny-pinching Rose found the women more satisfactory was in their willingness to work for less pay. McCormack paid his women microscopists a starting salary of $25. After a year on the job, they were taking home $40, or the starting salary of their male counterparts. The South Carolina state director, following McCormack's lead, used the $600 he had set aside to hire one man to employ two women instead. According to Rose, he was "delighted with the arrangement."[49] Shortly thereafter, Louisiana began to use women in its laboratory, and toward the end of the campaign Kentucky actually began to lend its women to other states.[50]

Throughout the difficult early months of organization, Rose freely admitted that he was feeling his way along from day to day. Aware of his inexperience in public health work but confident of the intelligence and ability of his initial appointments, he left his state directors alone to chart their own courses through the opening phases of the survey work. His openness to their suggestions – indeed, his dependence on them – heightened the sense of camaraderie and participation in policy formation and knit the group together in a way that certainly would not have been possible had Rose been working with a clear sense of direction. In a letter to Ashford which accompanied a copy of an early quarterly report, Rose put an optimistic front on the chaos he feared

Ashford would discover between the lines. "You will observe that these men are pursuing very different methods. It is our purpose to leave each to his own initiative for the present. Out of this variety of effort we shall expect by the survival of the fittest to come finally to a reasonably uniform method of operation."[51]

In policy matters concerning what he perceived as the proper relationship between the Commission and the states, Rose did not equivocate. His own natural reticence reinforced the lessons learned from the earlier experiences of the General Education Board. As the man with his hands on the purse strings from day to day, Rose was able to exert sufficient leverage on the state directors to bend them to a common standard in this regard. In theory, the method of disbursing funds was complicated. Each state director would submit a requisition for Commission funds, stating the specific purpose for which they were needed. Rose would present the petition to the Executive Committee, which would either turn it down or authorize Myers, the treasurer, to release the exact amount requested and to send it to the state board of health. The state board, in turn, would deposit the Commission's money in its own account and draw on it for the specific purpose given in the original requisition. As might be expected in an operation with which Rockefeller was associated, the accounting procedures of the Sanitary Commission were painstaking and thoroughly businesslike. Obviously, the Commission could not operate smoothly or efficiently if funds could not be disbursed without the permission of four men in three different cities. In actual practice, therefore, Gates allowed Rose to circumvent this unwieldy procedure by exercising his own judgment on the routine requests and shared with Rose the decisions on larger, more unusual ones. The Executive Committee, at its infrequent meetings, would rubber stamp Gates's and Rose's actions after the fact, and the Commission, at its annual meetings, would ratify all the decisions of the previous twelve months. Gates could rely on Rose's judgment in the normal course of events because the administrative secretary gave early evidence of sharing the chairman's narrow interpretation of the Commission's literal purpose—the eradication of hookworm disease in the South. For example, Rose declined on behalf of the Commission to underwrite the cost of postage for lobbying in support of an Arkansas public health bill by workers in the hookworm campaign, and he refused to grant Ferrell in North Carolina permission to use $2,000 to $2,500 to employ four or five county superintendents of health. When asked by the secretary of the California State

Board of Health for a contribution to combat hookworm disease brought into the West Coast by laborers imported from Asia, he demurred on the grounds that California was not in the South.[52]

If, however, through the mysterious workings of some multiplier effect, public health work in general benefited from the Commission's presence, then so much the better, as long as Commission funds were not specifically diverted to bring about this incidental consequence. Rose did not discourage the notion that the Commission sought to strengthen local public health efforts, but when questioned on this score, he would reply that the Rockefeller Sanitary Commission had been created for only one purpose—the eradication of hookworm disease in the Southern states. Only a major change in that policy would enable him to spend money for other things. His efforts to camouflage Rockefeller's connection with the work in order to limit the damage to the campaign from the philanthropist's wretched public image also worked to bolster the local reputations of the state boards of health. The state sanitarians themselves did not seem uncomfortable in the knowledge that their support came from a man widely regarded as a blackguard of the first order. They were happy to have money to spend for a change, whatever the source. James H. Cassedy has also suggested that "public health specialists, like other kinds of experts, were inclined to admire someone such as Rockefeller, who stood for efficiency in managerial methods."[53] But Rose was alive to the potentially damaging aspects of Rockefeller's association with the work, even if many of his field workers were not. He therefore suggested to the Arkansas state director: "I beg to advise that your office be styled, office of the Arkansas State Board of Health. I should think it might be well to omit all reference to the Rockefeller Commission."[54] Likewise, he counseled the Tennessee State Board of Health to leave the Rockefeller name off its stationery; "the letterhead should be your letterhead."[55] Whenever the question of title or attribution arose, he explained his reluctance to push forward the name of the Commission or its benefactor by noting: "We want to direct attention to the State Board of Health and create interest in it. This work is the work of the State Board of Health and all the people of the state should think of it as such."[56]

By the same token, Rose was sensitive to the fact that his Commission was especially vulnerable to the charge of meddling in local matters or dictating to local officials. He refrained from intervening in a squabble in Louisiana even when it looked as if this might lead to the peremptory dismissal of his hand-picked state director, a blow that would have seriously crippled the work there. In another situation, he refused to supplement the salary of the secretary of the South Carolina State Board of Health lest such a gesture should be interpreted as "undue interference" on the Commission's part.[57]

What little time remained in 1910 after the state campaigns had been organized was given over to a county-by-county canvass to determine the geographical distribution of the infection and the specific incidence for each infected area. The state directors initiated this survey with tours of personal inspection through the counties in which the heaviest infection was suspected. In these areas, they consulted with local physicians, visited the schools, and saw a few patients. When several contiguous counties were all found to be severely blighted, the state director designated the area a sanitary district and appointed one of the sanitary inspectors to take charge of the work there.

In conjunction with his preliminary survey, the state director sent out a series of letters to the doctors of the state explaining the work of the Commission and asking them to report the cases of hookworm disease they came across in the course of their practices. The first inquiries were persistently followed up with more letters and questionnaires. A disappointingly small percentage of physicians actually took the time to fill out the form and mail it back to the state director. Rose worried that the form might not be simple enough.[58]

Laboratory examinations of the stools of a few selected patients were performed and the results posted on a map of the state to give a visual representation of the geographic distribution of the disease. The conclusions reached as a consequence of this rather sketchy appraisal were genuinely alarming. Infection was demonstrated in 91 out of Virginia's 100 counties; in 97 of 98 in North Carolina; in 21 of 43 in South Carolina; in 108 out of 145 in Georgia; in 63 of 67 in Alabama; 65 of the 76 in Mississippi; and in Louisiana, after only two months' work, in 23 of 60 parishes. Forced to draw his conclusions without the benefit of a state laboratory, Olin West and his staff in Tennessee agreed that the infection was rampant in 52 out of 96 counties scattered all over the state. In North Carolina, where the able John Ferrell and a state public health service that was well developed by Southern standards got the work off to a quick and vigorous start, the state laboratory examined specimens from 5,556 people, taken by groups without regard to clinical symptoms. The representative samples included college students, soldiers in summer camps, orphans, and public school children. The results of the examinations indicated that 2,418, or 43 percent, were suffering from hookworm infection. The state directors, Ferrell included, led Rose to understand that in time, with more thorough surveys, the numbers would steadily increase.[59]

Using North Carolina's 43 percent infection rate as an indicator, Rose calculated that, of the 17,743,253 people in the nine states from which information had been gathered in 1910, fully 7.5 million might be victims of hookworm disease. They were scattered over 415,950 square miles, with about 80 percent living outside of cities and towns, in areas where the problem of soil pollution was most acute and where the victims were more difficult to reach. The officers of the Commission were shocked by the dimensions of the task before them, at least as suggested by the North Carolina figures. If Rose had been stingy with funds in the first year of the campaign, he would be even more so in the months to come. One million dollars, which seemed adequate in early 1910 when Stiles's best estimate of the number of sufferers stood at two million, now appeared too small in the light of a year's worth of evidence suggesting that there might be over three times as many hookworm victims as had been originally believed.

As yet, however, there was no reason to think that the North Carolina results gave a true impression of the disease's prevalence in that state, much less in the entire South: 5,556 people out of the 2,200,000 in the state represented a very small sample. Moreover, it could not even be concluded that this sampling represented an undistorted microcosm of North Carolina society, for several unavoidable biases belied the accuracy of the index. Almost all the people examined, for example, were under thirty. The North Carolina statistics were valuable in that they gave warning to the Commission and the field workers across the South that the job they all faced could conceivably be greater than they had previously thought likely. In fact, after lengthier and more comprehensive surveys, Ferrell's early returns proved high.[60]

While the county-by-county canvasses were still just getting off the ground, the Commission had already embarked on the second and third important aspects of the crusade—getting the victims cured and working to prevent reinfection. The state director and his staff followed three lines of attack in the early stages of the work in an attempt to reach the hookworm sufferers. They tried to enlist the assistance of the region's physicians, to get the people to seek examination and treatment, and to provide special help for the indigent.

In the long run, the most important of the three tasks was, unquestionably, winning over the doctors. If the South's medical fraternity would unite behind the efforts of the Commission, the other problems would become much easier to solve. Rose could see no other practical way of approaching the vast majority of hookworm victims except through the private practices of each state's physicians: "The State board of health in each State depends upon the physicians of the State to treat all cases of hookworm disease as it depends upon them to treat other diseases. This is a part of their practice; the State board would not take it from them."[61] At the inception of the campaign, there were 19,981 doctors in the nine participating states. Very few regarded the disease as a serious problem; fewer still could recognize on sight one of its victims. Rose, never one to approach a problem over-optimistically, reckoned that before hookworm could be driven from the field once and for all, every one of the twenty thousand physicians in the South would have to be alive to its dangers and treating its sufferers as a part of his normal practice.

The Commission, then, was embarking on a difficult task when it set out to win over the doctors of the South. As in other areas of its work, the Commission approached this problem from a number of angles. The state directors had already begun the effort with their personal visits to doctors in the sanitary districts and with the preliminary health letters and questionnaires. An estimated 16,512 such letters and circulars were sent to physicians across the South in 1910 alone. In addition to the personal correspondence, each doctor received regular mailings of official public health bulletins financed by the Commission but published by the state boards of health, which described the disease, cited medical references, and prescribed treatments: 49,066 bulletins were sent out in the first year of the campaign.[62]

The state directors, the members of their staffs, and officers of the Commission also delivered lectures and held demonstrations before the student body of medical colleges and at meetings of state, district, and county medical societies. Stiles reported attending meetings in nineteen states at which he delivered 122 addresses and clinics in 1910 alone. An integral part of these talks before professional as well as lay audiences, in addition to the microscopic diagnoses, was the lantern slide show. By the end of 1910, the Commission had distributed to the state boards of health 968 slides illustrating the anatomy and life cycle of the hookworm, the unsanitary conditions that encouraged its proliferation, the physical appearance of its victims, and its geographical distribution. Sets of some sixty slides were on file in the Commission's office to lend to any organization requesting one.[63]

If all else failed, the state directors were not above an appeal to the doctors' economic interests. Sidney Porter tried to reason along those lines with one recalcitrant physician in Pelican, Louisiana, while at the same time playing on his sense of honor:

"The poor are forever with us" and I feel that each physician from a stand point of humanity should give the people of his community such treatment as is necessary. Hook Worm disease, statistics show, decreases the earning capacity of the people from 50 to 65 percent, and I have no doubt that these people have been unable to pay you for services rendered for several years, but I believe if you will treat them for Hook Worm that it will relieve them of a condition that handicaps them, as I said before, by decreasing their earning capacity and they will be able to earn sufficient money to pay you for your services in the future. This should appeal to you from a business stand point if not from a stand point of humanity.[64]

McCormack employed the same tactics in a broadside to the physicians of Muhlenberg County, Kentucky, on the eve of a campaign there. "It is of special interest that every physician who has actively taken up this work has increased his income by so doing," McCormack pointed out. But lest Muhlenberg County's doctors conclude that he thought them bereft of the nobler impulses associated with the healing art, McCormack also suggested that the hookworm work offered a sublime opportunity to serve both interests at the same time: "Of course, it is the greatest thing to help the health of the people of our community but I am sure that it will be of interest to you to know that it will help you too."[65]

Although Rose privately expressed disappointment with the cooperation of the South's doctors at the beginning, these various methods of enlisting their support were moderately successful by the end of the first year. In his first annual report he was able to list approximately 3,400 physicians treating the disease, or about 17 percent of the region's medical force.[66]

Getting the people to seek examination and treatment presented the Commission's staff with more problems in the area of public realtions than the campaign to convert the doctors. Afflicted Southerners were so used to feeling weak and "out of sorts" that they had come to take their condition for granted. More often than not, they bristled at the suggestion that they were plagued by an unseemly parasite in their bowels. Clearly, the scientific, entirely professional line of attack used on the physicians would not work with all the people. They would have to be converted by more flamboyant, demonstrative methods. The sanitary inspectors conducted local sessions when they could, on the object-lesson principle of persuasion by specific example. The results of examinations conducted in the state laboratories were printed up and distributed by the sanitary inspectors. But the most ready form of access to the general public seemed, in 1910, to be the public schools and the colleges. After chapel exercises at the University of North Carolina, Ferrell asked the assembled students to volunteer for free examinations. The response was so heartening that he tried the same thing again at Wake Forest. All in all, some six hundred North Carolina college students agreed to be examined in 1910. Ferrell thought he detected an opportunity to take advantage of a snob factor that would come into play after his work with college students. "By making the idea 'fashionable,'" he wrote Rose, "among the better class of people the most highly infected class will be more easily reached and will seek examination and treatment." College students, by virtue of their social standing in their communities, would "prove to be unconscious workers for the cause during the summer."[67]

The work in the public schools combined actual examination of selected pupils obviously suffering from the disease with an educational campaign aimed at the public school hierarchies, from state superintendents of education down to the teachers themselves. Rose believed that in the schools was "a sort of key to [the] work in the states."[68] The method of approach was left to the discretion of the sanitary inspectors, but the state boards of health and the Commission provided them with leaflets or brochures designed especially for work in the schools. One Alabama physician reported that he always took a supply of such bulletins with him on each of his trips through the countryside. When he met a child exhibiting the symptoms of the disease, he gave him a copy, saying, "Show this to your mother and tell her I say I think you have that disease, and that you ought to see your family physician."[69] In June 1910, the Virginia State Department of Health printed a circular for distribution in the schools. On the front page, bracketed and in boldface type, appeared the following alarm: "Anemia of Hookworm in Virginia—It is scattered throughout the State; It weakens our people, saps their vitality; It decreases our productivity and burdens the community; It retards progress and befriends ignorance – It can be Cured and Prevented. This Bulletin Tells How."[70]

Most pamphlets of this sort were based on a model prepared by Stiles and produced in volume by the Commission's printers. Included in the brochure was a preface to schoolteachers stating the seriousness of the disease and asking for their cooperation:

Some of the teaching will involve a discussion of subjects not ordinarily mentioned in the schoolroom containing both boys and girls. *But human life is at stake, and in preparing this circular we must state facts in plain English; there is no escape from this method.*[71]

After the preface came a hookworm catechism ("Rule 1. Do not spit on the floor, for to do so may spread disease.") and a set of fifty-five questions and answers covering every possible facet of recognition, cure, and prevention including a Biblical justification for sanitary privies:

Question 3: Does the Bible warn against soil pollution? Yes; see Deuteronomy xxiii: 12 and 13: "12. Thou shalt have a place also without the camp, whither thou shalt go forth abroad"; "13. And thou shalt have a paddle upon thy weapon: and it shall be, when thou wilt ease thyself abroad, thou shalt dig therewith, and shalt turn back and cover that which cometh from thee."[72]

Interspersed throughout the question-and-answer section of the leaflet were drawings and photographs illustrating much of the same material covered in the lantern slides, but of a less technical nature. All in all, some 546,000 copies of this bulletin and others like it prepared by the various state boards of health were distributed during the year 1910.[73]

Perhaps because so many of the members of the Commission were well known and respected Southern educators, or perhaps because they did not see the Commission as a threat to their livelihoods or an implied criticism of their competence, public school teachers were more receptive initially to the hookworm campaign than the doctors. Since the schools were organized into districts, and the teachers took guidance from county and state superintendents as a regular part of their professional routine, they may also have been more suggestible than the Southern physicians. That they saw immediate and salutary changes in their pupils must have speeded their conversions as well. One schoolteacher in Loundes County, Georgia, wrote a letter of thanks to a field worker who had visited there shortly before, in which he marvelled at the "marked difference in the work of the pupils . . . They are cheerful and studious, now, where before they were peevish and stupid."[74]

Public lectures reached an estimated 196,000 people in the first year. In addressing popular audiences in his district, the sanitary inspector often had to drop his professional posture to assume the guise of the travelling storyteller. To intensify the lesson, he frequently showed slides of local conditions, with local landmarks prominently seen in the background. One inspector said his purpose in such lectures was "to make the story so simple, so direct, so vivid that every child will feel it tingle on the bottom of his bare foot when he walks on polluted soil."[75]

Most of the newspapers of the region that had been so hostile to the Commission at its inception made an about-face when enough facts were in to prove beyond a shadow of a doubt the need for a campaign against hookworm disease. Josephus Daniels, who had charged the readers of the *Raleigh News and Observer* not to "canonize Standard Oil Rockefeller" for his large gift to fight hookworm, came out with a four-column, illustrated story on July 21, 1910, stating that earlier skepticism had not been justified and calling for an all-out effort to stamp out the disease. Other editors and orators across the South quickly came to realize that the Yankee Dr. Stiles and his Rockefeller cronies were not intending to libel but preaching possible salvation. The Commission itself worked to bring about this reversal of attitude with a special campaign designed to win newspapers of the South over to the cause. The state directors' offices continually bombarded the editors with a barrage of articles publicizing the work of the Commission. Of the over 1,450 newspapers in the South, approximately 425 were personally visited by members of the state directors' staff. Papers in each of the nine states except Tennessee and South Carolina received over 2,500 letters from Commission officers and an estimated 646 articles for publication.[76]

Country editors, if they supported the Commission, did not scruple to run the Commission's press releases as if they were the papers' own editorials, which was exactly what Rose wanted them to do. The *Weekly Mercury* of Huntsville, Alabama, for example, featured pictures from the Commission's files in two front-page articles on December 4, 1912. In its own editorial, it praised the hookworm campaign as "an inspiring fight to the patriotic lover of America, for it shows how when philanthropist and scientist furnish the means and the knowledge how quickly American people, through their state and county government and by their individual efforts, will help to solve certainly a problem that was for centuries deemed unsolvable."[77] The editorial's headline, which appeared emblazoned on the front page under a picture of a school class in Washington County, Alabama, thundered, "Thousands of School Children Crippled in Mind and Body Through Activities of Hookworm." The second article in the same edition featured before-and-after photographs – supplied by the Commission to the *Weekly Mercury* – of a local family. "The tumbledown shack" in the first photograph was where "they all lived in misery, not knowing what was their trouble. They were illiterate." The second photograph showed a "neat two story house . . . where they all lived fifteen months after they were treated for hookworm disease. They were so restored in health and vigor that they set to work to make enough money to better themselves in every possible way." The third photograph depicted "the little white schoolhouse . . . where the children are now going to school to learn to read and write – things that were beyond the power and knowledge of their father and mother, their grandfathers and grandmothers, their great-grandfathers and great-grandmothers." The next-to-last photograph called the readers' attention to "the sturdy, healthy boy at the fence . . . one of the lads who are using their muscle and energy to bring the family into a prosperity never known before. He is industrious and capable now; but he was an invalid until he was relieved of hookworm disease." The final photograph was a portrait of the "family as it now is, well and happy and full of the new cheerfulness of clean and industrious living." The *Weekly Mercury* concluded by asking its readers, "Is it any wonder that this family is doing what it can to prevent the further spread of the disease? Is it any wonder that the father has built a sanitary privy and is observing those simple rules of sanitation that if generally lived up to would completely banish hookworm disease from the country?" The *Weekly Mercury*, photographs and copy furnished by the Commission, left little doubt regarding its own answers to these rhetorical questions.[78]

Rose himself had carefully orchestrated the effort to win over the South's newspapers. He proved to be even more sensitive than Page to the hair-trigger feelings of Southern editors. In refusing Page's offer to address the Round Table, a New York club to which Page belonged, Rose lectured his compatriot:

You know how sensitive our people are about having any man go to New York and talk about things that are being done in the Southern states. You know how much opposition was created in the press of the South by the publicity given to this work in the beginning. We have had to overcome. Everything is now going our way; all opposition is disappearing. I would not for the world do anything to interfere with the complete success of this work. For the present it is extremely important that the talking and writing be in the South from the state Boards of Health.[79]

To ensure that the press only reported good news, Rose carefully managed what was distributed for publication. When the state directors convened in Richmond in late September 1910, Rose recognized that a possibility existed for favorable free publicity. He warned A. W. Freeman, state director for Virginia and host of the conference, that "if the press is to be invited to any portion of the conference you ought to select your men, men that you could trust to publish what you want published and to keep out what you want kept out."[80] The first annual report of the Commission was a public document, and as such, fair game for the newspapers. The state directors could still exercise a modicum of control over how the publication of the report was covered, Rose felt, if the directors leaked the report to "one or two of the leading papers in each of the states," presumably ones that had already endorsed the Commission's activities. Once friendly newspapers had broken the story, "other papers will be apt to leave it alone." Rose urged is directors to "use your own discretion in this matter."[81] In that same annual report, and largely through efforts such as these, Rose could cite as cooperative the attitude of the press in each Southern state save recalcitrant Georgia and lukewarm Tennessee.[82]

Several state legislatures endorsed the work once it became apparent that it made good political sense to do so. The Attorneys-General of Georgia, Mississippi, and Arkansas first ruled that the counties of their states could not appropriate money for hookworm relief. A. G. Fort, the Georgia state director, reported that only an amendment to the state constitution could remove this legal impasse. In the meantime, he hoped the legal officers of Georgia would simply look the other way. The Mississippi state director persuaded the Attorney-General to reverse his decision after it had been called to his attention that Mississippi state law empowered the counties to vote money for the prevention of communicable diseases. W. S. Leathers, the state director, had little difficulty, once the statistics began to roll in from other states, in demonstrating that hookworm disease was indeed communicable. Altogether, eight states (Arkansas excluded) appropriated a total of $13,252.86 in 1910, or roughly one dollar for every three-and-a-half of the Commission's. The once-balky political hierarchy in Mississippi eventually swung enthusiastically into line. Vardaman wrote favorable editorials and sent a public commendation to Leathers and his staff. Vardaman's political under-study, Theodore G. Bilbo, endorsed the Commission; the speaker of the Mississippi House, a close friend of Leathers, worked actively on behalf of the hookworm campaign and personally introduced a bill designed to finance the collection of vital statistics; and the governor, Earl Brewer, hailed the Commission in his annual message. Other states may not have been able to boast of such spectacular political conversions, but after twelve months of operation, the Commission had won the support of the entrenched powers in the statehouses as well as in the fourth estate, except for a few pockets of resistance in Tennessee and Georgia.[83]

# 7

# The Days of Galilee:
# The Dispensary as Revival

Lack of uniformity in the maintenance of records made it virtually impossible for Rose to gauge the actual number of people examined and treated in the first year of the Commission's work. He did estimate that, up to the time of the publication of the first annual report, over 100,000 Southerners were examined for hookworm and approximately 42 percent of them were found to be infected. This was closer to Ferrell's early North Carolina returns than it was to Stiles's old estimate prior to the organization of the Commission. Of those found suffering from hookworm disease in the first year, 14,423 were on record as having received treatment. Rose well knew, however, that he could not trust the accuracy of these statistics. As yet, the work of the Commission on the local level had not been coordinated sufficiently to ensure that adequate records of treatment by both private physicians and field workers would reach the files of the state directors.[1]

With the publication of the first annual report, Rose felt that the time had come to establish a uniform system for gathering information and recording results. Accordingly, he brought his state directors together again in Atlanta on February 14 and 15, 1911, to devise a set of criteria they all could follow. They agreed that henceforth the degree of infection in a given county would be based on the microscopic examination of stool samples taken from a group of at least two hundred school children between the ages of six and eighteen. Every county in the South had schoolchildren who came from disparate social and economic backgrounds and by gathering under one roof for several months of the year simplified the field worker's task. In addition, by using schoolchildren as the common source for determining the degree of infection in the county, the Commission hoped to focus attention on the school and on the child. As Rose reasoned, "It is in the child that the home and the community are most interested."[2] Rose also noted that this type of survey, whether made with schoolchildren or any other population group, would supply the interested parties in the county with a precise, standardized body of information, furnish the basis of comparison with neighboring counties, and serve as the point of departure for a treatment campaign. By conducting the same kind of survey from time to time in the same county, health officials would be able to produce an up-to-date measure of the progress made in stamping out the disease in a given locale. By the time of the publication of the second annual report, surveys had been completed in 87 counties in the original nine states, resulting in degrees of infection ranging from 2.5 to 90.2.[3]

The year 1911 saw a broadening of the Commission's activities accompanied by the acceptance of this more precise method of keeping records. Rose, who soon found his original office too small for his expanded operations, moved to larger quarters. Kentucky joined the nine original states in the campaign, and primarily as a result of its active network of part-time county health officers, got off to a rapid start.

Another year's work on the survey of the distribution and degree of infection showed heavy incidence to be more widespread than previously estimated. (The table below gives some idea of the large geographical extent of the disease.) Of the 883 counties in these ten states, infection was found in 718 by the end of 1911; the remaining 165 had not yet been surveyed.[4]

Hookworm infection by county, 1910-1911.

| States | Counties surveyed by 1911 | Number of counties with infection | |
|---|---|---|---|
| | | 1910 | 1911 |
| Virginia | 100 | 91 | 93 |
| North Carolina | 100 | 97 | 99 |
| Georgia | 146 | 108 | 140 |
| South Carolina | 42 | 22 | 42 |
| Alabama | 67 | 63 | 66 |
| Mississippi | 79 | 65 | 77 |
| Louisiana | 59 | 23 | 27 |
| Arkansas | 75 | 20 | 57 |
| Tennessee | 96 | 52 | 95 |
| Kentucky | 119 | – | 22 |

A table of this sort, however, does not portray the degree of infection in a given area. One recorded case of hookworm disease was enough to throw the whole country into the ranks of the infected, even though under the new surveying procedures, one definite case would establish a rate of infection of only .005. Information from the field bore out Stiles's earlier hypothesis that incidence was heavier in the sandy coastal districts. Degree of infection was highest in North Carolina and Virginia through the tidewater areas, on the sea islands and along the coastal lowlands of South Carolina, in southern Georgia, and along the Gulf Coast in Mississippi and Alabama. Rose reported that in one county in the Gulf area, three public schools that he visited in succession produced 100 percent infection, including the teachers. In Tennessee, the heavier infection was demonstrated in the coves, on the slopes, and up to the plateau in the western part of the Cumberland mountain region. In Louisiana, hookworm was found to be most prevalent in the hilly regions in the northern parishes of the state, an early discovery that somewhat surprised the health officers there, who nevertheless reported to Rose that with a more extensive survey, their results would no doubt follow Mississippi's.[5]

Although Rose kept a close eye on the expenditure of funds to ensure that all monies spent went into the anti-hookworm work, he was quick to seize an opportunity to enhance the public reputation of the campaign without undue expense to the Commission. The Mississippi River rose in January 1912, overflowed its banks, and inundated the countryside for miles on either side in a five-state area from Kentucky to the Louisiana delta. Even without a flood to hold them up, the hookworm doctors had found the winter months to be the least productive. In the face of this natural disaster, no one in the Commission whose work had placed him in the river's path expected to get anything done. Rose took the opportunity to reap a harvest of good will by releasing his field workers in the five affected states to aid the Red Cross in relief work until the flood waters subsided.

With the support of the South's newspapers and public officials now fairly well established, the campaign began to gather a momentum of its own, apart from the public relations efforts, such as flood relief, of Rose and his state directors. Regional organizations, service groups, and businesses clamored to get into the act, now that the hookworm work had won the approval of the opinion makers and trend setters.

In at least four states—Virginia, Louisiana, Tennessee, and

South Carolina—the railroads offered to lend the Commission a hand. The Norfolk and Western invited Allen Freeman to join with spokesmen from the State Agricultural Department in a series of whistlestop tours across Virginia aboard the Better Farming Special. In addition to living accommodations, the railroad provided Freeman with space in a demonstration car for a hookworm exhibit and a model of a sanitary privy. Freeman called his work on the train "the most important I have done."[6] The Louisiana Board of Health also organized a Health Exhibit Train—two railroad cars that were hauled around from place to place free of charge by the more than thirty railroads operating in Louisiana. Sidney Porter, the state director, began travelling aboard the Health Exhibit Train as early as November 1910. By the beginning of 1911, he was writing Rose that as many as a thousand people a day were visiting his exhibit. "It is a physical impossibility to do any mental work here," he complained. "We work from sixteen to seventeen hours per day."[7] Tennessee also operated a health train for a year. While Stiles was conducting an investigation of rural schoolchildren in South Carolina, he, too, was given free use of a Pullman.[8]

Women's clubs across the South also lent their considerable support to the work of the Commission. McCormack noted that one of the incidental windfalls derived from his employment of young women in the state laboratory was the excellent impression it made on the women's clubs of Kentucky, which he called "the most powerful element behind us in our work."[9] The Arkansas Federation of Women's Clubs organized and staffed what amounted to a vigilance committee for hygiene and sanitation. A salutary interest in improving the standard of living in their respective communities no doubt inspired club women on a conscious level to cooperate with the Commission. And, by placing such a heavy emphasis on the crippling and retarding effects of hookworm disease on schoolchildren, the sanitary inspectors played on their maternal instincts and sense of responsibility to the rising generation. Those same Arkansas women, in addition to their policing activities, also sponsored a "Baby Health Contest" at the state fair to find "the most perfect baby in Arkansas." One of their number, Phebe Currie, put pen to paper in an effort to celebrate the occasion in poetry and capture the purpose of the competition. In her poem, a mother with a perfectly healthy baby boy of her own ("His dimpled arms, / His wealth of sunny hair") could not rejoice completely in her own good fortune because she was haunted by the spectre of other, less fortunate babies who, as a result of their mothers' ignorance, were not as well-tended as hers. ("From far-off heights of motherhood / 'Twas given her to see / How other babies, pale and sad, / Might healthier babies be.") The concerned young mother, no doubt a member of her local women's club, saw an ingenious way to get the simple message across to the less enlightened mothers of Arkansas. ("A contest plain and simple / Was the plan she did device, / For the caring of all babies / By hands both kind and wise.") That Christ would have approved of the "Baby Health Contest" Mrs. Currie did not for a moment doubt. ("For the 'Suffer little children' / Was to her a message true, / And what is done for these, the least, / Means all to me and you.")[10]

Almost everyone approved of the benevolent efforts of Southern ladies on behalf of "these, the least," but Flannery O'Connor did not. Writing in the early 1940s, she saw a different motive behind their apparently disinterested exercises in Christian kindness. Civic work of this nature, she believed, afforded the opportunity for socially ambitious women, trapped in sleepy, flyblown little towns, to scramble out of their humdrum existences over the bent backs of the cracker types conveniently at hand.

Social problem. Social problem. Hmmm. Sharecroppers! Miss Willerton had never been intimately connected with sharecroppers but, she reflected, they would make as arty a subject as any, and they would give her that air of social concern so valuable to have in the circles she was hoping to travel! "I can always capitalize," she muttered, "on the hookworm."[11]

Anywhere Southerners, whatever their social pretensions, came together—to learn, to pray, to eat, or to play—they found the young hookworm doctors of the Rockefeller Sanitary Commission. In Texas, where the campaign entered hard on the heels of the exiting Governor Campbell, the state director told of a traveling salesman, on a visit to a one-room schoolhouse in Steephollow, deep in the Piney Woods, who was peddling a book on wild animals. "What is the most dangerous animal in the world?," he asked the students. In one breath, several small children are supposed to have answered, "Hookworm!"[12] The editor of the High Point, North Carolina newspaper came back from the state fair to tell his readers that the two best things there had been the hookworm exhibit and the flying machine. The governor of Mississippi declared November 17, 1911, to be Public Health Day in Mississippi and urged the people to pause and contemplate what they could do to rid their state of hookworm disease. The schedule of events at the Chautauqua meeting in Demorest, Georgia, on the evening of August 20, 1912, included a lecture on "The Hookworm," complete with stereopticon pictures. McCormack reported that one zealous, if somewhat misguided, soul had sent to the state laboratory for analysis two ice cream buckets full of specimens collected at a county picnic in Buzzard, Kentucky. Unfortunately, the samples were hopeless mixed together and without identifying labels. At a revival in North Carolina, the preacher was persuaded to turn over one evening to two sanitary inspectors, one of whom lectured the faithful on the fly, the other on "Cleanliness is next to Godliness." Dozens of other examples illustrating the same point abound in the archives of the Rockefeller Foundation.[13]

Undoubtedly the most significant innovation added to the regular work of the Commission in 1911 was the county dispensary. Within a year, the dispensary method revolutionized the way in which the Commission got people to seek treatment. The first dispensary established in the South specifically for the treatment of hookworm disease was opened by Dr. John C. Culley in Columbia, Mississippi, on December 17, 1911.[14]

Culley, a recent graduate of the Vanderbilt medical school, signed on as a sanitary inspector in the Mississippi campaign on August 20, 1910, and was assigned to the sanitary district that included Marion County. Columbia, a town of some two thousand people and the county seat of Marion County, lay in the gently rolling, pine-covered hills of south-central Mississippi, on the Gulf and Ship Island Railroad line midway between Gulfport and Jackson. By 1910, the timber resources of the area had been pretty well played out, and most of Marion County's 23,500 people lived in poverty while they struggled through the transition from lumbering to agriculture. Although the incidence of hookworm disease in the Columbia area was staggeringly high, few people could afford to seek treatment. The news of this local affliction had not come as a surprise to Marion County doctors in 1910. At least two of their number had been treating the disease for seven years.[15]

Charles C. Bass, just out of medical school at Tulane, happened to be passing an open lecture room at a meeting of the American Medical Association in New Orleans in 1903 when he heard Stiles's voice and decided to drop in to listen. Stiles, of course, was talking about hookworm disease, and Bass, who later wrote a textbook on the subject, realized for the first time that the government zoologist was describing with eerie precision the appearance and the behavior of most of the children in the rural areas around Columbia, where he had recently established a practice. Before leaving New Orleans, Bass bought a microscope. Within days of his return to Columbia, both he and his partner, Dr. Hector H. Howard, later to become a field worker for the Rockefeller Sanitary Commission and the International Health Commission, were treating their patients for hookworm disease.[16]

Culley did not have to begin his work in Columbia, then, by persuading the local medical establishment of the presence of hookworm disease in their midst. The political establishment, however, was a different matter. The county health officer, Dr. A. D. Simmons, agreed to allow Culley the use of several rooms, a hall, and a lavatory in his office building, but Culley needed funds from the county, or from someone, to buy medicine and furnishings. When he first approached the Marion County board of supervisors with a request for an appropriation of $300 to buy thymol and outfit his little clinic, he was rebuffed. Not one to be so easily dissuaded, Culley fell back on guile when it appeared that frankness would not win over the politicians. "I went out and collected specimens of feces from the sons of the members of the board," he wrote. "I placed these specimens in warm containers until the larvae hatched. I then placed these larvae under the microscope which I had set up in the court house and asked each member of the board to look."[17] When the board of supervisors reconvened to consider Culley's request a second time, no one cast a negative vote. W. S. Leathers, the Mississippi state director, noted in a regular report to Rose, dated December 7, 1910, "Dr. Culley is now working in Marion County, at Columbia, and I received a telegram from him to-day saying that the Board of Supervisors had on yesterday appropriated the necessary money for buying medicines in that county."[18]

Rose had seen hookworm clinics in operation in Puerto Rico that closely resembled Culley's dispensary, but he and Ashford had agreed that the Southern farmer was much too obdurate and fiercely independent to seek help from a clinic in his neighborhood, even if encouraged to do so. It was with some skepticism that Rose awaited the first returns from Columbia, although he refrained from expressing his reservations once the men in Mississippi had decided that the experiment was worth a try. The Columbia dispensary was so remarkably successful from the moment it opened its doors — perhaps because Bass and Howard had helped to prepare the way — that Rose was able to write in his first annual report less than a month later: "The dispensary is running

at its full capacity and hundreds are being turned away for lack of
facilities. This is the most promising move that has been made in
the direction of supplying treatment for the indigent."[19] Rose
paid Culley a visit in early 1911, and came away a believer. "I
must confess," he wrote Leathers, "that the way people are taking
hold of this is a revelation to me. I had no idea that the people
would come in for treatment in such numbers."[20] At Rose's insistence, the Commission appropriated $180 to pay the salary of
a trained nurse to run the dispensary for three months while Culley traveled about the countryside and made arrangements for a
second dispensary, this one at Brookhaven in Lincoln County. By
the end of May 1911, Culley's original dispensary had given out
1,744 treatments to approximately 1,000 individuals, all at a cost
to Marion County of $92.50, or about 18 cents per treatment. The
backbreaking schedule implied in the statistics took its toll of
Culley's health. A stomach ulcer forced him out of the hookworm
work in May 1911, and into the quieter, more orderly life of a general practitioner in Oxford, Mississippi, where he numbered the
Faulkners among his patients.[21]

With Rose's strong encouragement, other states quickly took
up the dispensary work. By the time he came to write the second
annual report, Rose could draw on practical experience from all
over the South to revise his estimate of the dispensary's value:
"In its surprising development during the present year we have
almost ceased to think of it as a means to supply treatment to the
indigent in view of its incomparably greater value as an agency
for teaching all the people by demonstration."[22] The wider deployment of dispensaries brought only minor changes in Culley's
method. Each dispensary came to be established for a definite
amount of time, and each was moved from place to place within
the county according to a publicized itinerary.

Apart from its crucial role in getting the victims of the disease
to seek attention, the hookworm dispensary deserves special consideration for the manner in which it incorporated several aspects
of life in the rural South at the turn of the century into the work
of the Commission. In this respect, the hookworm dispensary
borrowed from its institutional predecessor, Seaman Knapp's
farm demonstration program. In effect, a well-run dispensary
skillfully merged the primary medical and educational objectives
of the Commission with a wealth of local custom and tradition.
The entire campaign in the South, as a result of the introduction
of dispensaries into its regular routine, was cast in a less foreign,
much more congenial light.

In many important ways, the county hookworm dispensary resembled an old Southern tent revival. First, the sanitary inspector would go into a community and confer with members of the local power structure—the mayor, councilmen, leading business figures, educators, clergy, newspapermen, and doctors. From them he would secure pledges to support a dispensary in the county for several weeks. As a rule, too, the county would appropriate a sum of money, anywhere from $50 to $300, to help with the financing. The sanitary inspector and his assistants would then blanket the county with posters and circulars announcing the dates and locations of the dispensary. A typical dodger used in this intensive advertising campaign contained inducements such as these:

There will be illustrated lectures and demonstrations on sanitation daily. These will be in plain simple terms that any one can understand and any one can also see the working of that wonderful instrument, the microscope, by simply asking the man in charge . . . Many of the bad feelings people have, are due to hookworm and we have found that about half the people are infected . . . THIS IS ABSOLUTELY FREE—THE STATE AND COUNTY ARE PAYING FOR IT . . . Come out on the dates named and see what is being done. Don't think it is the other fellow who needs this. It may be you.[23]

Regular announcements were run in the newspaper; employers persuaded their workers to attend; preachers exhorted their congregations.

When the opening day came around, people from the town and its outlying farms turned out *en masse* to greet the dispensary. Rose marveled:

The people came in throngs; they came by boat, by train, by private conveyance for 20 and 30 miles. Our records contain stories of men, women, and children walking in over country roads 10 and 12 miles, the more anemic at times falling by the way, to be picked up and brought in by neighbors passing with wagons. As many as 455 people have been treated at one place in one day. Such a dispensary group will contain men, women, and children from town and country, representing all degrees of infection and all stations in life. A friend who had just visited some of the dispensaries said to me recently: "It looks like the days of Galilee."[24]

Interestingly enough, when seeking to convey the spontaneous excitement that greeted his farm demonstration program, Knapp had also spoken of "the power which transformed the humble fishermen of Galilee."

Dr. Benjamin E. Washburn's description of a typical North Carolina dispensary on opening day is worth studying. He had just joined the work of the Commission a few weeks earlier, and was accompanying Dr. Platt W. Covington, an experienced sanitary inspector, to watch and to learn. The community was Mills' Spring, a small town in the North Carolina mountains with a population of less than 8,000 including the surrounding countryside; the dispensary was to be held on the grounds of the local schoolhouse.

By the time of our arrival the men had moved the benches from the schoolroom and arranged them under the large oak trees in the yard. Tables had been placed for the dispensary exhibit and for the microscopist, and more than a hundred specimens had already been brought in. On another table were bottles containing worms which had been recovered from patients following treatment.

Covington was a master at handling a crowd of this kind. First he got the microscopists started at their task. Then he called up people who had received treatment . . . and interviewed them. All declared they had received great improvement; and the doctor listened to each one's chest with his stethoscope, presumably to determine if his heart was improved. This procedure was called "sounding" by the people.

Treated patients having been seen, the doctor next gave a lecture. He stood on a box and held a set of charts to which he pointed as he talked. On the way to Mills' Spring he had told me of two rather old and rather large ladies who always sat on the front seat. [Covington had conducted dispensaries before in Mills' Spring.] These ladies were on hand . . . Just as Covington had told me, when he explained the effects of hookworm disease on children, how it stunted their growth mentally and physically and left them ignorant and incapable of earning a decent living, the old ladies got out their handkerchiefs and began wiping their eyes. This was soon followed by subdued sobs and finally by copious tears.

By the time the lecture was over the microscopists had examined a number of specimens. Persons found positive were called up to receive their treatment.

The exhibit was next explained to the crowd and, again, it was told how hookworm disease is spread through soil pollution and by flies, dirty food, contaminated water from open wells, and unprotected springs; and it was emphasized again that typhoid and other bowel diseases are spread in the same manner. After the bottles of hookworms had been passed through the crowd, a demonstration was made with ascaris. This was always more impressive to the crowd since these large round worms, sometimes twelve inches in length were widespread in this mountainous section and familiar to everyone.

The demonstration over, Dr. Covington asked if a Sunday School singing leader was present. There was; and a lean tall man came forward with a tuning fork. After sounding a few "do do re re's" he led the crowd in "Onward Christian Soldiers." This was followed by other church songs and the singing continued for perhaps half an hour. By this time the microscopists had more specimens to report upon. The doctor made another lecture, the fat old ladies crying as before, more treatments were dispensed and another demonstration was made. By this time it was midday. The different families went to their buggies or wagons to eat the lunches they had brought. This meant that the sandwiches we had brought ... were supplemented with delicious fried chicken, freshly made biscuits, boiled eggs, and with pound cake and stewed peaches for dessert.

The crowd had not diminished by the afternoon as other persons and other families came to take the places of the ones who had been examined and treated during the morning. Many, however, had come prepared to spend the day, and did so. The dispensary continued through the afternoon and it was nearly five o'clock before all the specimens had been examined and the necessary treatments dispensed.[25]

The several parallels between the mechanics of dispensary work and a tent revival are evident in Washburn's account. Like the revival, the dispensary was a temporary, almost itinerant event, sweeping into the town for a few exciting days before disappearing. Both were preceded by several quiet conferences with the town dignitaries to enlist their permission and support; both enjoyed large advance promotional campaigns. North Carolina went so far as to hire someone fulltime—a Mr. R. O. Self—to act as an advance agent in charge of all the preliminary arrangements for a county dispensary. On the big day the townspeople and country folk turned out in their buggies and wagons, dressed in their Sunday finest. By Charles Grandison Finney's day, at least, it was generally believed that a good revivalist could "work up" a revival on his own initiative, without waiting for a divine signal. Likewise, it was up to the sanitary inspector to determine if conditions in a community were right for a dispensary. As the success of a revival depended on the skills of the evangelist, so did the dispensary rise or fall with the ability of the doctor in charge. In order to rivet the attention of their audiences, both the revivalist and the sanitary inspector resorted to gimmicks, some of which took advantage of the people's technical ignorance, and all of which played on either their emotions or credulity. The revivalist called on sinners who had seen the light and been saved to come forth and proclaim their salvation before the congregation. Covington, working on the same principle, summoned former sufferers who had taken the cure to join him in front of the audience and be interviewed. If the word of these witnesses was not good enough in itself, Covington added medical punctuation to their stories by "sounding" them with his stethoscope. Evangelists harangued their terrified (and enthralled) congregations with fiery images of hell and eternal damnation; the sanitary inspector caused old ladies to sob with vivid stories of the malevolent parasite's effect on little children. Both constantly reiterated simple themes: the revivalist called for repentance and salvation, the doctor, for treatment and prevention. Both also relied on the electrifying effect of on-the-spot conversions. The man of God incessantly referred to the good news revealed in the Scriptures, but his symbols were often more tangible things such as a roaring fire or, as in some parts of the Appalachians, a poisonous snake. The sanitary inspector, on the other hand, derived his special authority from "that wonderful instrument, the microscope" – the Gospel according to Bausch and Lomb – but he used as his visual aids simple charts and bottled worms, no matter if they were not hookworms so long as they were large enough to impress the audience. When it came time for a change of pace in both the revival and the dispensary, the leader called on the people to join in the singing of a few gospel songs. In the free time between sessions, whether at a revival or a dispensary, the audience broke out the box lunches and had a picnic.[26]

The architects of the hookworm dispensary may not have had this obvious model in mind when they worked out the details, but the comparison was not lost on at least two of the sanitary inspectors. One, in Alabama, after an especially successful day at a dispensary, wrote to the state director that, "One might almost talk of today as a sanitary revival."[27] In Kentucky, thousands of whose citizens had gathered at Cane Ridge over a century earlier to trigger the Second Great Awakening, another sanitary inspector noted to McCormack, "It is like a big, old-time camp meeting."[28] In the same letter, he reported his conversation with an old farmer who had approached him on one of the last days of a dispensary in Jefferson County: "Doctor, after I heard your lecture Wednesday night I went home and rolled and tumbled all night; could not sleep for thinking how unclean I have lived and am living now." The field worker sent him home, mind at rest, with instructions on how to build a good outhouse – from "anxious seat" to privy seat with the absolution and best wishes of the sanitary inspector.

A kind of missionary fervor pervaded most successful dispensaries but perhaps never so much as at another one in Kentucky. McCormack told of how one of his sanitary inspectors, J. S. Lock, rode alone on a mule for several days over the Cumberland Mountains into the remote hollows of Harlan and Leslie counties, both "entirely off ordinary lines of travel." So isolated were these mountain districts before the advent of coal mining that McCormack wrote Rose, "These people are aboriginal Anglo-Saxons and I am reliably informed that in many places they are still speaking sanscrit."[29] Lock was met with rifles at the ready, but he proved to be a master of tongues. In whatever language they spoke, he quickly made converts of the suspicious mountaineers, who had never seen a camera, much less a microscope. That they endowed his hookworm dispensary with a quasi-religious significance is best borne out by one of Lock's photographs, which shows a wedding held, at the request of the couple, in his dispensary.

The dispensary, then, added an important dimension to the work of the Commission. It not only carried the campaign to the people of the South as never before but also translated its message into a language and a ritual that they could readily appreciate. The success of the dispensary is echoed in the statistics. In his final report on the Commission's activities, in which he summed up the full five years' work in the South, Rose noted that 578 counties had expended $90,366.46 for the maintenance of dispensaries. In the course of their work, dispensary microscopists had performed 1,087,666 examinations at an average cost of eight cents per examination. Doctors had treated 440,376 people at dispensaries, at an average cost to the county of twenty-one cents for each treatment. This absolute number of hookworm sufferers treated in dispensaries across the South represented approximately 69 percent of the total number of people treated anywhere, at any time, during the five-year period of the Commission's existence—a surprisingly high percentage in view of the fact that the dispensary did not become an integral part of the campaign until fairly late in 1911, well into its second year.[30]

Rose and Gates succumbed to a preoccupation common to revivalists, with results that some felt were harmful in the long run to the overall anti-hookworm campaign. For want of a better index, the revivalist tended to judge the relative success of his latest revival by counting the number of self-professed converts and comparing the total to previous harvests. Little if any effort went into an attempt to ascertain how many of those expressions of faith were genuine and long-lasting and how many were merely spontaneous emotional outbursts, born in the heat of the moment and forgotten almost as soon as the revivalist folded his tent and left town. Rose, too, fell victim to the attraction of the raw statistics issuing forth from the dispensaries. He turned a less than sympathetic ear to the occasional state director, like West in Tennessee, who pleaded, out of fairness to the field workers, that Rose take into account the widely different circumstances from state to state. West feared, with some justification, that the administrative secretary had come to regard the number of people examined and treated in a given dispensary as the primary indication of the sanitary inspector's efficiency. A crude body count, in West's opinion, did not take into consideration factors such as the degree of infection in a community (and the related degree of interest in a dispensary), the political climate, the support or indifference of the local doctors, the power and influence of the state board of health, and a host of other peculiarities that could determine the outcome of a dispensary. Freeman in Virginia argued that in areas of low infection an elaborate dispensary was a waste of time. Rose, however, continued to pour money into the dispensary program and to pit doctor against doctor in a kind of frenzied competition to roll up the numbers. He regularly published and distributed among the state directors lists that ranked the field workers according to the number of examinations and treatments in dispensaries. In the fourth annual report, he included a section entitled "Records Made in County Dispensary Work." He also snatched especially productive sanitary inspectors out of their home districts and sent them around to the less successful states as troubleshooters, a practice that rankled the state directors who were supposed to benefit from the outside assistance. Gates, always the good manager, also became mesmerized by the reports flowing from the dispensaries, especially those that pointed up the cost effectiveness of the dispensary system.[31]

Stiles did little to increase his influence with either man by calling into question the value of the dispensary results. As early as August 1912, he warned Rose: "The more I go around the country where clinics have been held the less importance I am able to attach to the statistics of the clinics. I have seen family after family where they tell me they have visited the clinics, had been told they had hookworm disease, had taken the medicine home, but were afraid to take it." Stiles said he would be surprised if more than half the people given the thymol actually swallowed it. "I do not mean to discourage the clinics," he concluded, "for they are doing good advertising, but I am more and more convinced as time goes on that their curative value is overrated."[32] Rose agreed that too much medicine was thrown away surreptitiously, but he did not think as much was wasted as Stiles claimed. At any rate, he argued, "the dispensary has not been organized as an agency for the final cure of the people."[33] Its value lay more in its educational and demonstrative potential. He put the scientific secretary on the defensive by pointing out that as soon as a hookworm purge as effective but not as dangerous as thymol was developed, the incidence of unswallowed medicine would fall precipitously.

Rose's last point was well taken. Thymol was a most effective vermifuge, but to many who endured its side effects, the cure must have seemed worse than the disease. A dosage that was concentrated and large enough to dispatch the parasites was also unfortunately potent enough to nauseate the host. The hookworm doctors worried less, however, about a few upset stomachs than they did about the ever-present possibility that one of their patients would die from the treatment. They lived constantly with the unsettling knowledge that they were dispensing a potentially lethal drug to people who were unused to following the instructions of a physician. Moreover, they were unable in most cases to supervise treatment personally. Although the sanitary worker could diagnose a case of hookworm disease in a few minutes at the dispensary, he could not treat it on the spot. The best he could do was to admonish the patient, send him home with a handful of dangerous capsules, and hope that the instructions were followed.

The instructions were relatively complicated and the regimen of treatment, a nuisance. The North Carolina state director has described it:

The patient should take little or no supper on the evening before the thymol is to be administered. As early at night as is convenient he should take a dose of Epsom salt. The next morning as early as the salt has acted, half the number of capsules of thymol prescribed for the whole treatment should be taken. Two hours later the remaining capsules should be taken. Two hours after the second dose of thymol, another dose of Epsom salt should be taken, which will expel the hookworms that have be enforced to loosen their hold on the intestinal wall by the action of the thymol, and will also get rid of the excess of thymol before it has had time to produce any harmful effects on the patient. Nothing should be eaten on the day the capsules are taken until the final dose of Epsom salt has acted well.[34]

Despite the confident assertion that the second dose of Epsom salts would prevent the disquieting effects of the thymol on the patient's system, many who underwent treatment later complained of nausea, dizziness, and weakness. A good meal no doubt would have alleviated much of the giddiness and loss of strength, but a good meal, Southern style, would likely have killed the patient.

As alcohol and oils dissolve thymol, making it actively poisonous to the patient, the use of them in any form would be exceedingly dangerous. Gravy, butter, milk, all alcoholic drinks and patent medicines, which generally contain alcohol, should be forbidden on the evening before and on the day of the treatment.[35]

"The more I think of it," Stiles wrote, "the more I am impressed with the risk the field men have to assume."[36] He himself narrowly avoided tragedy on at least two occasions. What he once took to be a potbellied, preadolescent girl with an advanced case of hookworm disease turned out to be a pregnant woman. Had she taken the thymol Stiles was on the verge of sending her home with, she would surely have lost her baby. On another occasion, he had to take away a bottle of "chill tonic"—laced with alcohol—from a patient who, understandably enough, wanted to chase the obnoxious taste of thymol. "I may be altogether too conservative," he wrote, "but my conservatism is increasing rather than decreasing and I sincerely hope that in the dispensary system we will not have any accidents."[37]

Stiles might have helped to allay his own fears by coming up with a less dangerous alternative to thymol. Eventually he did, but his chenopodium with alboline substitute came too late to change the method of treatment used throughout the life of the Sanitary Commission.[38] Southerners did violate the strictures on diet, and occasionally their negligence cost them their lives. Stiles "heard of several deaths during treatment [for] hookworm disease," and Ferrell reported the death of a child in Halifax County, North Carolina. Rose, reluctant to credit hearsay damaging to the Commission's reputation, did not keep statistics on thymol-related deaths. To verify the accuracy of each story would, in his opinion, have deflected his hookworm doctors from their primary responsibilities. In retrospect, it seems unlikely that rural Southerners would have turned out in such large numbers at the dispensaries if it was widely believed that the sanitary workers were peddling death. Ferrell claimed that the people in Halifax County placed the blame on the parents, not on the dispensary.[39]

Exonerating the men of the Sanitary Commission from culpability in the death of a child was one thing; taking the medicine oneself after hearing reports of what it could do was something altogether different. Who would know? Stiles had good reason to question the amount of thymol that was actually swallowed. He suggested that Rose might at least modify the nomenclature in the annual reports so that the category in question would be entitled "Number of Persons to Whom Medicine Was Dispensed," rather than "Number of Cases Treated." In the "Explanatory Notes" of the third annual report, Rose called his readers' attention to the fact that some people undoubtedly did not take their medicine, but he quickly added that "the number of persons who have thus failed to take the treatment is more than offset by the large number of persons who get treated by physicians and otherwise of whom no report is received and no record made."[40]

Much of Rose's optimism and Stiles's pessimism can be attributed to their different professional backgrounds. Rose, a conscientious teacher and a good progressive, shared with John Dewey, another progressive educator, the sanguine belief in the infinite educability of mankind toward a more enlightened, well-regulated society. To Rose, hookworm disease was a problem not unlike illiteracy—a remediable impediment to a richer, more satisfying life. Stiles, on the other hand—the son of a Methodist minister before he became a medical scientist and public health official—knew only too well that mankind was depraved, that individuals would invariably harm themselves if left to their own devices. To Stiles, hookworm disease was a symbol of man's filthiness: as long as there existed a way for people to catch it, they would.

As their difference of opinion suggests, Rose was temperamentally predisposed more toward one aspect of the Commission's work, and Stiles to another. Rose, infatuated as he was with the ephemeral results of dispensary work, understood the long-range importance of attacking the disease at its source—soil contaminated by people with unsanitary habits. But he felt it more important for the time being for the Commission to demonstrate convincingly that hookworm sufferers could be cured. Once restored to health with the Commission's help, the former victims would be more likely to adopt the methods suggested by the sanitary inspectors to guard against a recurrence. The rest of the community, seeing the transformation in the lives of their neighbors, would join them in the work of prevention. Stiles placed much less faith in the ability or the inclination of people to act as voluntary agents in their own regeneration. They could, however, be coerced into stamping out the disease. A small, elite corps of public health officials, if given the authority by municipal and state ordinances and the necessary funds from tax revenues, would see to it that the people built privies and took their medicine whether they wanted to or not.

Soon after the creation of the Commission, Stiles was at work trying to design a cheap, effective outhouse. He could easily justify this project to both his employers.[41] The Sanitary Commission, for obvious reasons, placed a high priority on the development of a sanitary privy that most people could afford. The Surgeon General also recognized that many serious public health problems other than hookworm disease—typhoid fever and contamination of water supplies, for example—would be greatly alleviated if people stopped answering the call of nature wherever it was made.

The same conference of state directors that had adopted a set of guidelines for determining the degree of infection in a county also ratified a uniform plan for conducting a sanitary survey in each state. At the same time that a field worker and his microscopist were visiting a community for the first time and examining its schoolchildren, they would also inspect at least one hundred rural homes and record the privy conditions on a six-point scale from A (for the best, most sanitary) to F (for no privy at all), assigning an index number for each class. Stiles classified the privies in the following manner:

| *Class* | | *Index no.* |
|---|---|---|
| A. | Water carriage or Marine Hospital Barrel (LRS) | 100 |
| B. | Watertight and rigidly flyproof privy | 75 |
| C. | Watertight, closed in back, not rigidly flyproof | 50 |
| D. | Closed in back, surface privy | 25 |
| E. | Ordinary open in back surface privy | 10 |
| F. | No privy at all | 0 |

To calculate the sanitary efficiency of a county, the field worker would multiply the number of privies in each class by the index number for that class, add up the totals, and divide the grand total by the total number of homes. The sanitary index for one sample county was then estimated as follows:

| 1 | B home at | 75 | 75 |
|---|---|---|---|
| 2 | D homes at | 25 | 50 |
| 165 | E homes at | 10 | 1650 |
| 58 | F homes at | 0 | 00 |

The total index number (1775) divided by the total number of homes (226) yielded 5.19, giving county X a sanitary index of 5, in round numbers, on a scale of 100.[42]

Rose's hypothetical county was in worse shape than most Southern counties, but not by much. In the fifth and final annual report, Rose noted that the Commission's agents, between 1911 and 1914, inspected 250,680 homes in 653 counties, for an average of 383 homes per county. The sanitary index for all the homes visited over the four-year period was only 6.3 percent. In other words, half the homes inspected had no privy at all, and nine out of ten privies found at the homes that could boast one of some sort were of the most rudimentary, least sanitary kind.[43]

State sanitarians and members of the Commission alike agreed that only a massive privy construction program would secure the temporary gains won in the dispensaries. Sewage systems were out of the question in rural areas and small towns. Water closets, septics tanks, and privies were the only solution, but of all the available alternatives, which struck the best balance between sanitation and cost? Stiles and two of his colleagues at the Marine Hospital in Wilmington, L. L. Lumsden and N. Roberts, developed the LRS privy—named for the three of them—which consisted of two water-tight, connected barrels beneath floor level and zinc-lined box above. No one found fault with the LRS privy on sanitary grounds; it was by far the most effective system of its kind yet devised. Its construction cost, however, placed it well outside the means of most Southern farmers. Far more realistic was the pit privy, which could be made safe enough if dug according to certain specifications and periodically filled and relocated. Stiles would not compromise, arguing instead that "in view of present-day knowledge" about the transmission of diseases, the LRS privy was "the least that can possibly be demanded."[44] Other designs might cost less to build, but Stiles steadfastly maintained that to sanction their construction would be to indulge in a false economy. As a public health official he could not bring himself to acquiesce in a scheme to save the farmer a few dollars at the risk of his health. A marginally safe privy might be better than no privy at all, but Stiles refused to lend the weight of his own reputation to a policy of practical compromise. He remained adamant throughout the years of his association with the Commission, although most of his colleagues came to accept the trade-off sooner or later. Ferrell, first in North Carolina and later as Rose's assistant at the Commission headquarters, sanctioned the construction of pit privies as a matter of course, a policy that Stiles vehemently, if impotently, attacked. "I do no propose," he fumed, "to become a party to any ten cent mining stock pseudo scientific campaign such as Doctor Ferrell carried on in the South under the name of the Commission."[45] For the record, Ferrell discreetly avoided an open collision with Stiles by refusing to recommend one model over another. He cautioned the Arkansas state director that "there is such a divergent [sic] of opinion on the subject that I do not think it worth while to endorse any one type of closet too strongly." He fell back, instead, on the principle of caveat emptor. "My own method has been to put before the laity the principles we are advocating and let them use their own discretion in the details."[46]

A few communities opted for the LRS privy. Haynesville, Louisiana, a town of a thousand people, passed an ordinance requiring that all privies within its boundaries conform to the features of the Stiles model. A tax of forty cents per month was levied on each household to establish a fund out of which scavengers were paid to collect the refuse and assistance provided to upgrade existing closets. McCormack and his associates in Kentucky developed a modified version of the LRS privy that amounted to a concrete septic tank. In the summer of 1915 alone, more than two thousand Kentucky sanitary privies were built. Freeman's model privy, part of his exhibit on the Better Farming Special, was of the LRS type. Indeed, whenever a sanitary inspector included a privy in his demonstrational apparatus, it was always a class A model, generally based on the Stiles design. C. H. Brownlee, a Texas field worker, built a model sanitary privy in the yard of the courthouse in every county in which he conducted a dispensary, and left it there when he moved on. F. L. Routh, of South Carolina, went Brownlee one better. On the outhouse he built in front of the Laurens County courthouse, he hung a sign which read: "Build a privy now—use it always; It is cheaper than a coffin."[47] In New Albany, Mississippi, a community club of 800 "earnest" women (so styled by their president) established as its only membership requirement the obligation to construct a sanitary privy. Polite society in the rural South had come a long way since the days when Stiles was threatened with bodily harm for broaching the subject of outhouses in his public addresses.[48]

Despite the enthusiasm with which it was taken up in some parts of the South, the privy construction program lagged behind other Commission projects. Rose lamented the fact that "it has been more difficult to get improvement in sanitation than to get the people treated."[49] Ferrell privately observed, "Our work in installing sanitary privies has not, on the whole, been so satisfactory as in the treatment of infection."[50] The county dispensary only asked that the farmer sacrifice one day to the sanitary inspector (no real sacrifice for someone whose tedious daily routine made any distraction an event) and that he take the thymol free of charge. We have already seen that many – perhaps upwards of one-half of those to whom medicine was dispensed – threw it away. To get the same farmer to return home and build a privy on his own initiative and with his own money and labor proved far more difficult. Even the most rudimentary outhouse – a ramshackle lean-to over a hole in the ground – betokened a significant change of habit, a level of commitment that the dispensaries, for all their excitement, did not require.

When he was first setting up his General Education Board programs in the South, Buttrick had found it necessary to walk very gingerly around the vexed question of race. Rose, faced with an even more delicate public relations problem, had also to watch his step. As early as 1902, Stiles had observed that Southern blacks did not appear to suffer as much as whites from the more severe ravages of hookworm disease. "The negro race," he concluded, "had this disease for so many generations in Africa that it has become somewhat accustomed to it."[51] But, lest anyone take this to mean that the Rockefeller Sanitary Commission could ignore the racial problem, Stiles went on to point out that their greater immunity made blacks better carriers and spreaders of hookworm infection. Their African forbears had over centuries worked out an ecological détente of sorts with the hookworm; Southern whites enjoyed no such truce. Stiles argued that "the white man owes it to his own race that he lend a helping hand to improve the sanitary surroundings of the negro."[52]

In the tense atmosphere of race relations in the early twentieth century, Stiles's reasonable assessment was discarded by polemicists and self-appointed experts on race who nevertheless seized on his evidence to blame Southern blacks for what they saw as

yet another act of treachery. In a *McClure's Magazine* article entitled "The Vampire of the South," Marion Hamilton Carter argued that "Negro crimes of violence number dozens where his
sanitary sins number tens of thousands. For one crime a mob will
gather in an hour to lynch him: he may spread the hookworm and
typhoid fever from end to end of a state without rebuke."[53] It is
not clear from this passage, at least, whether Carter believed the
hookworm or the black to be the greater "vampire," or whether he
thought lynching the proper punishment for black "sanitary
sins."

Another remarkable piece of racist billingsgate entitled "The
Health Menace of Alien Races" appeared in *The World's Work*.
Perhaps Page may be excused from sanctioning its publication,
for when it appeared, he had been in London for several months.
The author, Dr. Charles T. Nesbitt, began with Stiles's observa-
tions but quickly moved on to a theme of his own.

In 1902, Dr. Stiles discovered that the hookworms, so common in Africa,
which are carried in the American Negroes' intestines with relatively
slight discomfort, were almost entirely responsible for the terrible plight
of the Southern white. It is impossible to estimate the damage that has
been done to the white people of the South by the diseases brought by
this alien race ... As this phase of the race problem continues to be
studied, it is unevitable that further investigation will produce still
stronger evidence that the races cannot live together without a damage
great to both; so great, that even now the ultimate extinction of the
Negro in the United States is looked upon by many as assured.[54]

The descendants of the victims in the great historical kidnapping
were apparently to be held accountable for the lesser crimes that
followed from the original abduction, and Stiles's small fund of
scientific information was being used in the preparation of the bill
of particulars.

Although Rose did not foster the racist tirades and pseudo-
scientific arguments, neither did he raise his voice in public contradictions. He offered quiet encouragement to his state directors
who came to him with proposals of their own for carrying the
campaign into black schools and communities, but invoked the
principle of nonintervention when called upon to employ the
financial clout of the Sanitary Commission to force work toward
that end. He was not stretching the truth when he wrote in 1912
that:

The work done thus far in all the states has been, as I understand it,
without any race distinction. The field men have visited the schools for

both races; have lectured to audiences of both races; literature is sent to physicians, teachers and people of both races; the state laboratory is giving free examination of all specimens sent it without regard to race; the dispensaries examine and treat all people that come regardless of race. I have never visited a dispensary without seeing both races present. One of the fine things about this to me is that the work has been done without any suggestion of race distinction.[55]

These were claims that few other Southern-wide organizations could, or would want to make in 1912. But Rose refused to push the point. Two years earlier, Ferrell mentioned that a black physician had applied for a position with the Commission in North Carolina and tried to coax Rose into seeing the advantages of such an appointment. One of his arguments was that "the salary and travelling expenses of such a man would not have to be as much as is paid to the white Field Agents."[56] Still, Rose equivocated. He later privately agreed that "it is probable that in the course of time some special work will have to be developed among the negroes . . . Just what form this will take I cannot foresee. The Commission will, of course, expect each state to work this out its own way. The Commission does not take the initiative in any matters of this kind . . . As to the advisability of having a negro physician in the field, that must be worked out by the state Board in each state."[57]

No black doctor ever found employment with the Sanitary Commission. The number in private practice who responded to Commission mailings by treating their own patients is not known. There are a few indications that other organizations, using other sources of funds, at least looked into the problem of hookworm infection among blacks. For example, the National Medical Association in 1910 appointed a committee to study the question and appointed Dr. John A. Kenney of Tuskegee Institute as the chairman.

Since the white field workers had been chosen in large part on the basis of their compatibility with the white laymen they would be expected to serve, it is not surprising to learn that, in the absence of specific guidance from Commission headquarters, they oftentimes reflected the fears and prejudices of the society from which they came. A circular prepared by a Mississippi field worker and distributed among the "leading farmers and planters" of Winston County illustrates the point.

The Negro race is to some extent immune to the evil effects of the Hook Worm disease, but they are not immune to the infection which is very high in this country. Their Habits, their ways of living, and their environments, are all favorable to the spread of the disease among their own race, as well as its transmission to the white race. The negro cannot be interested in, nor can they readily understand the situation. They cannot be reached through regular channels, yet unless they are reached, treated and cured, they will continue to infect the soil and perpetuate the disease among the whites.

So, for self protection, every PLANTER WHO HAS NEGRO TENANTS, EVERY PERSON HAVING NEGRO SERVANTS, EVERY COMMUNITY HAVING NEGRO FAMILIES LIVING NEAR THEM, should induce these negroes to seek treatment at once.[58]

Isolated pieces of information do indicate that some work was carried out specifically in black groups and communities. The evidence, however, is scant. The white superintendent of the Virginia Colored Insane Asylum took it upon himself to use funds from his operating budget to treat all the 1,500 inmates in his custody. Rose hailed his efforts as "the largest bit of work that has been done in the way of treating the negro race."[59] After he had settled Wilmington, Stiles wrote of his eagerness to begin work in the black churches. Garrison of Arkansas reported to Rose that he had helped to arrange "for Dr. J. H. Barabin, colored, to visit the colored institutes. I secured a pass for him and he volunteered his services to deliver lectures on sanitation, hygiene, hookworm disease, etc., and a colored carpenter, capable of drawing blue prints and thoroughly competent in every way, is to follow Dr. Barabin and demonstrate the method of building sanitary closets . . . Fortunately it will be at no expense for the Commission."[60] A year later, Garrison recounted the details of a meeting in New Orleans. "Quite a number of prominent colored representatives were there and it would have surprised you to have listened to some of their papers."[61]

The few surveys conducted exclusively among black groups produced ambiguous results. In 1911, Ferrell, after examining "500 to 750 negroes," found the rate of infection to be only one-third as high as that for a comparable group of whites. Despite the inexplicable imprecision of his sampling technique, his data seemed to bear out Stiles's 1902 contentions. In Grimes County, Texas, however, a 1913 survey revealed a contradictory pattern. Of the 1,841 whites examined, 533 (29 percent) were found to be infected as against 155 of 246 blacks (61 percent). In neither survey was any indication given of the relative severity of infection.[62]

If the Texas and North Carolina figures demonstrated anything, it was that much more work needed to be done before any sound comparative generalizations could be made. Rose did not urge his field workers to gather information by race. "Personally," he argued, "I see no particular reason for race distinctions in the sanitary survey."[63] His annual reports remained faithful to that conviction. Nowhere in the welter of graphs, charts, headings, and subheadings was race used as an evaluative criterion. From this distance in time and with the figures Rose and his field workers have left us, it is impossible to estimate the number of Southern blacks examined and treated by agents of the Sanitary Commission. Rose kept to himself his reasons for discouraging racial distinctions in the surveys. He was a prudent man, and he no doubt wanted to avoid unnecessary controversy of any sort. He was also a Southerner, sensitive to the cluster of emotional associations that adhered to the subject of race. Finally, he was a humane man, and he had seen how Stiles's value-neutral data from 1902 had been unscrupulously employed for ideological purposes. As the administrative secretary of the Commission, he could ensure that statistical information based on race would be put to innocent, even praiseworthy purposes within his own organization. If it were to be published, however, he could not control the ways in which it might be interpreted by race-baiting polemicists. For whatever reasons, Rose chose not to gather it at all.

The slow-going pace of privy construction brought home to Rose the limitations of his beloved dispensary program in a way that Stiles's warnings had not. Since he had always regarded the dispensaries primarily as educational devices, perhaps he did not view their failure to obliterate hookworm disease as a limitation. In any event, after four years of hard work, Rose could not point to one village or county in the South that the Commission had helped to rid of the parasite. If the Rockefeller Sanitary Commission were to begin to live up to the promise inherent in its name, its members and its employees would have to be prepared to settle down into a protracted, far less glamorous routine of quiet effort in every county of the South for many years to come. In late 1913 and early 1914, the indications were that Rose and his state directors had begun to make the transition from dispensary work to something more enduring. The Commission began actively to encourage the state boards of health to develop conditions conducive to the appointment of full-time county health officers. In addition, Rose authorized the inauguration of an intensive community program in a handful of small towns in order to demonstrate that hookworm disease could be eradicated in a given locale if enough effort were brought to bear. It was true that four of the five years allotted to the Commission under the terms of Rockefeller's original gift had already elapsed, but Rose felt sure that the work would be extended. Only two-thirds of the $1 million had thus far been expended. At the annual meeting of January 1914, no one from the Rockefeller offices brought up the question of the Commission's life span when five of the members, including Stiles, were re-elected for new three-year terms. John Ferrell had been brought up from North Carolina to give Rose the technical and administrative help he had never had before, a move that would make little sense were the Commission going out of of business on schedule. The force of field workers had been augmented by the addition of fifteen new physicians in 1914. These men must have had some assurance that their jobs would last for more than a few months. The General Education Board had been originally chartered for a finite amount of time, but Rockefeller had always extended it, using the occasion of each extension as an opportunity to increase its endowment. John D. Rockefeller, Jr. was known to favor continuing the hookworm work in the South even though it would mean approaching his father for a second appropriation. Finally, everyone associated with the Commission had come to understand that the real work of eradication had yet to get really under way.

Rose and his doctors had good reason to believe that 1914 would see the continuation and expansion of their campaign, and that when 1915 came, their programs would still be active and in place. They were all shocked and dismayed when Gates – the man who had insisted that the word "eradication" be included in the Commission's title – pulled the rug from beneath them by abruptly and unilaterally terminating the work and disbanding the Commission at the end of its fifth year.

# 8

# "Henceforth Thy Field Is the World": From Sanitary Commission to Rockefeller Foundation

In 1908, during his first meeting with Stiles, Gates had called the suggestion that he support an anti-hookworm campaign in the South "the biggest proposition ever put to the Rockefeller office," but by early 1914, he had completely lost interest in the Sanitary Commission. All indications coming out of the states after four years of work there led him to believe that the dispensaries had outlived their usefulness—that the "days of Galilee" were over and only the tedious business of mopping up remained. Impatient by nature, he did not welcome the prospect of overseeing such plodding work for years to come. The mercurial pace and the dramatic results of the dispensaries better suited his temperament and more closely fitted his notion of what an outside philanthropic agency should do. Moreover, two things in 1913 had encouraged him to cast his restless eye beyond the South to places where the hookworm was still entrenched and unopposed—places that were as much in need of the blitzkrieg tactics of the dispensary program as the South had been four years earlier. In May 1913, the Rockefeller Foundation had been chartered—its mission "to promote the well-being of mankind throughout the world"—and three months later, colonial officials in London had invited the Foundation to extend the anti-hookworm work started by the Sanitary Commission into the colonies and territories of the British Empire. These two events had served to work a revolution in Gates's sense of the immediately attainable. After the British invitation, the South seemed very small indeed.

Raymond Fosdick devoted two chapters in his history of the Rockefeller Foundation to a careful discussion of the chain of events leading up to its creation. He noted that Gates and the two Rockefellers first started mulling over the idea of a foundation as early as 1905. In a letter dated June 3, 1905, Gates invited the elder Rockefeller to direct his thoughts to the just claims of posterity on "this great fortune of yours." Since the "moral responsibility" for its accumulation rested with Rockefeller, and not his heirs, he must also, by virtue of an "inexorable logic," bear the moral responsibility for its deployment. "If you and Mr. John are, therefore, to discharge this trust while you live, there is only one thing possible to be done, and that is to provide funds in perpetuity, under competent management, with proper provision for succession, which shall be specifically devoted to the ends of human progress." This grand system of interlocking funds

should be so large that to become a trustee of one of them is to make a man at once a public character. They should be so large that their administration should be as much a matter of public concern and public inquiry and public criticism as any of the functions of government are now. They should be so large as to attract the attention of the entire civilized world, their administration become the subject of the most intelligent criticism of the world, and to their administration could be addressed, both directly and indirectly, the highest talent in those particular spheres of every generation through which the funds should go, to the remotest ages of mankind.[1]

Gates was calling for a philanthropic organization to stand in relation to Rockefeller's individual charities in much the same way as Standard Oil did to the more than forty separate companies under its hegemony. Different human problems would require different philanthropic solutions, which in turn would call into being special programs, each with its own board of directors, but all would fall under the rubric – and under the control – of the Rockefeller Foundation. By late 1906, there were indications that Gates and the two Rockefellers had begun to think in terms of one "trust" along the lines of Standard Oil, rather than of a series of distinct "funds." On December 31, 1906, in a New Year's Eve letter to his father, Rockefeller, Jr. brought up an earlier conversation in which they had discussed the creation of "a large trust to which you would turn over considerable sums of money to be devoted to philanthropy, education, science, and religion." He wondered "whethered it would be possible to get together a single group of men who could be expected to have knowledge and interest along so many different lines." His minor reservations notwithstanding, the younger Rockefeller was eager to press forward with their plans.[2]

By 1909, the year in which Stiles first gave his hookworm demonstration in Gates's office, the elder Rockefeller was ready to act. On June 29, two months before Stiles was invited to address the Lake George meeting of the Southern Education Board and four months before the creation of the Sanitary Commission, Rockefeller signed over 72,569 shares of Standard Oil stock (worth $50 million) in a deed of trust to Gates, his son, and Harold McCormick, his son-in-law and heir to the International Harvester fortune. No public announcement accompanied the gift, and Rockefeller reserved (and later exercised) the right to rescind it at his own discretion. The three trustees were instructed to petition "the Congress of the United States, or . . . the legislature of such state as they deem advisable, for a suitable corporate charter."[3] Accordingly, on March 3, 1910, as Rose was getting settled into his Washington office and preparing for his trips to Florida and Puerto Rico, Senator Jacob H. Gallinger of New Hampshire introduced in the United States Senate a bill to incorporate the Rockefeller Foundation. Fosdick has noted that the 1910 bill was virtually identical to the charter of the General Education Board, obtained without difficulty by the same process. Fosdick also observed: "There were distinguished precedents for this kind of procedure; between 1889 and 1907, thirty-four organizations had secured incorporation by the United States, including the Carnegie Institution of Washington, the American Academy in Rome, and the American Historical Association."[4]

Actually, no federal or state law required that Rockefeller seek a public charter before setting up the Foundation. Jerome D. Greene, general manager of the Rockefeller Institute at the time of the hearings, discreetly pointed out during one of the Congressional sessions on the bill that the simple deed of trust, already transacted, would suffice. After all, it was Rockefeller's money to do with as he saw fit. By seeking a charter, Starr J. Murphy told a Senate Committee, Rockefeller was offering Congress an opportunity to ensure that the fund would "always be used for the public welfare and for no other purpose."[5] Implicit in the offer was the warning that if it refused to issue a charter, Congress would be relinquishing control over an organization that was destined to appear in any event.

Far from anticipating a fight, Rockefeller and Gates hoped that a charter from the United States Congress would lend an aura of prestige to their enterprise. Their petition, however, achieved the opposite effect by calling down the obloquy of prominent men both in and out of government. As one study of the charter proceedings put it, "The idea that John D. Rockefeller meant well was still greeted with skepticism."[6] The petition to obtain a charter for the Foundation created another forum – this time, the Senate of the United States – from which Rockefeller's critics could voice their skepticism. Senator Hoke Smith of Georgia took his lead from his voluble constituent, Bishop Warren Candler, in denouncing the bill on the grounds that Rockefeller's pernicious philanthropic meddlings, as seen in the General Education Board and the recently created Sanitary Commission, were almost as reckless and troublesome as his business ventures. Others smelled various rats. "The papers," Fosdick recalled, "rang with such phrases as 'the kiss of Judas Iscariot,' 'the Trojan horse,' and 'tainted money.' "[7] The journalist John Temple Graves, writing in the *New York American*, compared Rockefeller to Jean Valjean in Victor Hugo's *Les Misérables*. Both men had led early lives of crime, Graves observed; both had escaped into virtue and beneficence. In the United States of 1910, society played the part of Hugo's Sisters of Mercy – forgiving the criminal and lying to the police. "This," Graves concluded, "is a forgiving age."[8] The United States Attorney General, George W. Wickersham, was not cut out to play a Sister of Mercy. He warned President Taft: "Never has there been submitted to Congress, or to any legislative body, such an indefinite scheme for perpetuating vast wealth as this; and personally I believe it to be entirely inconsistent with the public interest that any such bill should be passed."[9] Taft agreed and joined in condemning "the proposed act to incorporate John D. Rockefeller."[10] American Federation of Labor President Samuel Gompers noted derisively, "The only thing that the world could gracefully accept from Mr. Rockefeller now would be the establishment of a great endowment of research and education to help other people see in time how they can keep from being like him."[11]

In retrospect it seems obvious that Rockefeller and Gates had completely misread the public mood, or at least that they had overestimated Congressional immunity to it. Their charter petition was ill advised in every respect. Although Rockefeller was certainly accustomed to public vilification, he had not taken accurate note of the degree to which hostility to him had intensified in the seven years since the General Education Board charter bill sailed through Congress. He and Gates certainly noticed each separate attack, but they misgauged the cumulative effect on his already blackened reputation. Since the General Education Board had been created in early 1903, the attacks had increased in frequency and intensity. In early 1905, for example, Washington Gladden, the best known Congregationalist of his day, had openly castigated his church's Board of Foreign Missions for accepting a gift of $100,000 from Rockefeller. "Is this clean money?" he asked. "Can any man, can any institution, knowing its origins, touch it without being defiled?"[12] Gladden's attack backfired, but its effect remained. If not for the first time then surely by the most illustrious public figure to date, Rockefeller's charitable activities had been called into question.[13] His business practices had certainly come in for their share of criticism over the course of his career, and although he had ostensibly retired, the controversy surrounding his name failed to abate. Whatever his official status in its boardroom, Standard Oil was still very much in business, and Rockefeller would be forever linked in the public mind with the corporation he had created. Ida Tarbell's inflammatory history of the Standard began to appear in *McClure's* as early as 1902, but it was not until 1904 that it was published in book form. Americans in the first decade of the twentieth century, whipped into a state of high dudgeon by muckrakers like Tarbell on the one hand and by the showy anti-trust suits of Roosevelt's Justice Department on the other, were outraged to see the worst of the "malefactors of great wealth," the man whom Robert La Follette called "the greatest criminal of our age," escape time and again the sanctions of the law, his fortune not simply intact but steadily mounting, keeping ironic pace with the national ire. Progressive hopes rose briefly in 1907 when Judge Kenesaw Mountain Landis found Standard Oil guilty, under the terms of the Elkins Act, of 1,642 separate counts of price fixing and imposed a fine of $29 million. But those same hopes were dashed when Landis' decision was overturned on appeal. It later came to light that Rockefeller's close confederate, John D. Archbold, had in 1900 bribed Ohio Senator Joseph B. Foraker, an opponent of Taft for the Republican presidential nomination in 1908, with $15,000 for services rendered in the defeat of a Senate bill judged inimical to the interests of Standard Oil.[14]

Despite the reversal in the Landis case, the federal government continued to stalk the conglomerate. The Justice Department renewed its assault in the courts almost immediately – this time in the Missouri federal circuit court – with a suit calling for the dissolution of the trust itself on the grounds that it represented a conspiracy in restraint of trade. The government won its case in Missouri, won again in the appellate court, and in early 1910 prepared to present its argument once again, this time before the United States Supreme Court.

Through it all, Rockefeller himself maintained a scrupulous and outwardly serene silence. He rarely granted interviews; rarer still were his public responses to accusations in the press. When called upon to testify in court or before a legislative investigative committee, he was courteous under questioning, cautious and precise in his answers, and unflappable. He volunteered nothing and always claimed to have acted out of the best of motives and according to the highest standards of conduct. His "Random Reminiscences," serialized in Page's *World's Work*, also conceded nothing and revealed little. The image of himself that he chose to present for public scrutiny was of a plodding, warmed-over Poor Richard, but without Franklin's wit, inventiveness, or underlying sense of irony.

His apparent legal invulnerability and his righteous disregard of criticism galled his critics all the more. Although he shunned publicity until well into the 1920s, Rockefeller received more press coverage in the first decade of the twentieth century than any other public figure except Theodore Roosevelt. Perhaps no other American of his day was so despised. How is one to account for the antipathy he inspired? Other men – Carnegie, for example, or J. Pierpont Morgan – were almost as rich, and yet they did not incite the public to fury as Rockefeller did. Several other multi-millionaires of his generation – Harriman, Frick, and Gould among them – had moved just as ruthlessly to their fortunes. Even after the historian has taken into account the normal degree of hostility mixed with grudging admiration displayed toward any extraordinarily wealthy man by citizens in a democracy ostensibly based on the principles of free enterprise, he is still left with the task of explaining the extra measure of outrage reserved for Rockefeller alone. It is especially incumbent upon the student of the Rockefeller Foundation and its related philanthropies to try to understand it, because it impeded their operation to a significant extent.

Perhaps a key to an explanation lies in the pious aphorisms of "Random Reminiscences." Rockefeller may well have inspired the hatred of his fellow citizens because they sensed that at heart he was too much like them. He may well have been regarded as abhorrent precisely because he was not aberrant. Carnegie certainly bore little resemblance to the average American of his day: a Scottish immigrant and a self-proclaimed agnostic, he was widely believed to uphold the bleak, cheerless principles of his friend Herbert Spencer. Morgan was a suave, cultivated Machiavellian who lived in a Renaissance palace in midtown Manhattan. Frick collected Italian art. Vanderbilt, at the opposite extreme, had seemed to revel in his reputation as a cutthroat. But the case of

Rockefeller, the richest of them all, was different. There was certainly no denying that Standard Oil reached into virtually every
home in the land and touched the lives of millions of Americans in
a direct and obvious way as U.S. Steel and the House of Morgan
did not. Rockefeller's representatives drove their kerosene wagons down the streets of American communities everywhere. Still,
the larger part of an explanation of the resentment he provoked
lies in the fact that he sprang from the same matrix of values as
most white, middle-class, native-born Americans—values which
he never abandoned. On the contrary, he steadfastly credited the
old verities with his success. The self-confessed and proud prod-
uct of a commonly revered configuration of home truths, Rockefeller—through the very act of building Standard Oil, and later
defending it—had not so much perverted those values as suggested their bankruptcy in the modern age. Faith in the Protestant God, devotion to family, hard work, attention to detail,
thrift, sobriety, and the importance of competition in character
formation: if adherence to these principles had built Standard Oil,
then might not Ragged Dick himself someday become a threat to
the commonweal? Few reformers in the progressive era advo-
cated a wholesale reworking of the American economic system;
fewer still proposed that the code of beliefs undergirding it be
abandoned. By tinkering a bit here and there with the mechan-
ism, they hoped to guard against— or at least to control—the occasional interloper, the cynical manipulator, who would subvert
it. But Rockefeller professed to have arisen from deep within the
substratum of values that supported and nurtured the very system itself. His career paradoxically cast suspicion on the fundamental tenets that most Americans—he and his critics alike—
proudly claimed as their birthright. Ideally, from the point of
view of his enemies who shared his faith in the old ways, Standard Oil would collapse like the House of Atreus from a hidden
flaw in its construction, or in the character of its patriarch. In
1910, however, nothing seemed less likely. To destroy his empire
in the courts would be a step toward rehabilitating those values,
but not enough in itself. Rockefeller must also be proved a hypo-
crite. And so his enemies watched, biding their time, while his
critics in the press reported his every action.

There were several who saw in the timing of his huge public
benefactions an indication of the most sinister kind of hypocrisy
at work. A $32 million gift to the General Education Board had
come at the time of the Landis decision. Gallinger had introduced
the Rockefeller Foundation charter bill just five days before the

Standard Oil attorneys were due to file their briefs with the Supreme Court. More than one businessman in the preceding fifty years had come to regret the day he had trusted Rockefeller; more than one prosecutor who thought he had Standard Oil on a legal hook had seen it wriggle through a loophole and escape. On the face of it, the offer of Congressional control over the proposed Rockefeller Foundation looked safe enough, but too few Senators were willing to accept the idea that Rockefeller was acting in good faith. In the past he had finessed state legislatures with ease. If that was what his legal wizards were up to now, the Republic would be the one left holding the bag. The man who had invented a new definition for the word did not inspire trust in a majority of Senators. Although passed by the House of Representatives, the charter bill, despite several restricting amendments (all accepted by the Rockefellers) failed three times to clear the Senate. The Senators were no doubt bolstered in their opposition by the Supreme Court's decision in March 1911 to uphold the order of the lower court dissolving Standard Oil.[15]

When it appeared likely that the charter bill would encounter heavy resistance in Congress, Rockefeller had written, "I feel increasingly that even in order to get the charter we should not commit ourselves to any definite specific line of work. This hookworm enterprise can be used effectively as illustrating the kind of thing such a charter would make possible."[16] Accordingly, Jerome Greene, who orchestrated the lobbying in Washington, held up the record of the Sanitary Commission as an example of the humanitarian activity the Foundation could be expected to pursue. By January 1913, repeated frustrations at the hands of his opponents in Congress had forced Rockefeller to relent on his decision to avoid a definite commitment. Before the final vote in the House of Representatives, Greene pledged that the Foundation's first order of business would be the continuation and extension of the work of the Sanitary Commission. Headquartered in Washington, Rose and his administrative assistants found themselves drawn into Greene's lobbying efforts. For a short time in 1912, Greene tried to mobilize Rose and the politically influential physicians on his payroll in an assault on the stubborn members of the Southern Congressional delegation. Allen Freeman, state director in Virginia, was placed in charge of a pro-charter letter-writing campaign among the Commission's field workers, who were also encouraged to promote the bill back home in the Congressional districts. Whether their efforts helped to ease the bill through the House cannot be determined. It is clear, however, that Greene and his employers considered the work of the Sanitary Commission one of their strongest weapons in the charter fight – so strong, in fact, that of all Rockefeller's benefactions, many of which were much larger, only the Sanitary Commission was singled out for special mention in this way.[17]

After the 62nd Congress adjourned in March 1913, leaving the charter bill hanging in the Senate, Rockefeller and Gates decided to abandon the fight in Washington and turn instead to a more compliant (if less prestigious) state legislature. If they had been unable thus far to secure their charter under a Republican administration, what chance would they have once Wilson and the 63rd Congress took office? Within weeks of the Congressional adjournment, the much less suspicious legislators of the New York Assembly passed an act of incorporation, without encumbering amendments, which was signed into law by the governor on May 14, 1913.

After incorporation had been obtained, Rockefeller's advisers moved quickly. With $35 million in stock at their immediate disposal (and another $65 million within a year), the trustees of the new Foundation[18] met on June 27, 1913, to approve the preamble and resolutions – drawn up by Gates – establishing the first major subdivision of the philanthropic empire under their control and the first to be set up under the terms of the charter. The organization was to be called the International Health Commission,[19] but the resolutions which formally called it into being read like a summary of the Sanitary Commission's work in the South:

WHEREAS the Rockefeller Sanitary Commission, organized in 1909 for the eradication of Hookworm Disease in the United States, has found more than two million people in the Southern states to be infected with the disease, involving vast suffering, partial arrest of physical, mental and moral growth, great loss of life, and noticeable decrease in economic efficiency over vast regions; and

WHEREAS the Commission has treated or caused to be treated more than five hundred thousand persons; has ascertained that the diagnosis of the disease can be made with ease and certainty and that it can be readily cured and easily prevented; has found that the people, physicians, state boards of health, county and municipal officers are eager to cooperate in all helpful ways, and that, following the treatment and cure of this disease, an intelligent public interest is awakened in hygiene and in modern scientific medicine and in practical measures for permanent public sanitation . . .

Thus far, the resolutions of the new Commission could not be distinguished from an optimistic litany of the old Commission's accomplishments. Only in the third paragraph did the trustees move on to a recitation of the goals they had set for themselves.

WHEREAS the Commission has ascertained by diligent and extensive inquiry that Hookworm Disease prevails in a belt of territory encircling the earth for thirty degrees on each side of the equator, inhabited according to current estimates by more than a thousand million people; that the infection in some nations rises to nearly ninety percent of the entire population; that this disease has probably been an important factor in retarding the economic, social, intellectual and moral progress of mankind; that the infection is being spread by emigration; and that where it is most severe little or nothing is being done towards its arrest or prevention; therefore be it
RESOLVED that this Foundation is prepared to extend to other countries and peoples the work of eradicating Hookworm Disease as opportunity offers, and so far as practicable to follow up the treatment and cure of this disease with the establishment of agencies for the promotion of public sanitation and the spread of knowledge of scientific medicine.[20]

To the casual student of the Foundation reading over the resolutions establishing the International Health Commission, it would appear that the success of the Sanitary Commission in the South had prompted the trustees to extend the work around the world. In fact, the accomplishments of the Sanitary Commission only confirmed in Gates's mind a course of action he had already tentatively established almost a year before Culley opened his first dispensary. A clue to Gates's earlier thinking is to be found in the first clause of the third paragraph of the resolutions: "the Commission has ascertained by diligent and extensive inquiry that Hookworm Disease prevails in a belt of territory encircling the earth." Rose had conducted that "diligent and extensive inquiry" at Gates's request, as one of his first assignments as the administrative secretary of the Sanitary Commission. In April 1910, less than three months after Rose's first Atlanta conference and only a few weeks after the introduction of the Foundation charter bill, Gates obtained permission from the elder Rockefeller to ask Rose to make a preliminary survey of the prevalence of hookworm disease around the world. Gates himself later wrote that, following his first meeting with Stiles in 1909, his "imagination began to play around the alleged devastation and suffering caused by this disease."[21] Ashford's Puerto Rico evidence and the results of Gates's own private inquiries in 1909 reinforced Stiles's contentions. Knowing that Rockefeller had already secretly signed over $50 million in a deed of trust as seed money for a philanthropic foundation with a global mission, Gates must have been thinking of a world-wide campaign as early as 1909, although he gave no indication to Stiles or to anyone else at the time that he was contemplating anything more than a program to combat the disease in the South.[22]

Rose put together a questionnaire and circulated it, with the assistance of the State Department, through American consulates around the world. A year later, he published the results of his survey in the Rockefeller Sanitary Commission's Publication Number Six, *Hookworm Infection in Foreign Countries*. Responses from 54 countries had helped him to compile a profile of a disease so ubiquitous and so entrenched that a philanthropic organization on the scale of the inchoate Rockefeller Foundation would be overmatched. Stiles's estimated two million Southern hookworm victims represented only 1/500th of the potential sufferers in a broad zone running around the globe on either side of the equator from 30 degrees south latitude to 36 degrees north. Over half of the world's population lived in this hookworm belt, much of it concentrated in the territories and possessions of the United States overseas holdings and of the various European colonial empires.[23]

Gates was anxious to begin a global anti-hookworm campaign, but he could not proceed as long as the Foundation remained unchartered. In the two years between the appearance of *Hookworm Infection in Foreign Countries* and the New York Legislature's act of incorporation for the Rockefeller Foundation, the dispensary program in the South had demonstrated, to Gates's satisfaction at least, the feasibility of a massive but relatively inexpensive program against hookworm disease. If the results of the Sanitary Commission's work in the states had not planted in Gates's mind the original suggestion for a much larger undertaking, nothing in its career between 1910 and 1913 caused him to question his earlier decision.

Woodrow Wilson, no doubt unintentionally, facilitated the launching of the International Health Commission. By the time the twelve members of the new Commission, eight of whom were carry-overs from the older one,[24] were ready to act, the new president had installed one of their own, Rose's old friend Walter Hines Page, as the Ambassador to the Court of St. James's. Rose, the newly deputized director-general of the International Health Commission, had anticipated the need for the cooperation of the British colonial authorities and had sent a copy of *Hookworm Infection in Foreign Countries*, at the time of its publication, to the British ambassador in Washington. Two years later, when he was finally prepared to make overtures in the direction of the Colonial Office, Rose was delighted to find one of his staunchest allies strategically placed in London. In late June 1913, he wrote to Page, asking for his opinion on the advisability of a trip to England. Two weeks later, on July 14, Page cabled, "Everything ready. Come."[25]

With Ferrell in Washington to direct the daily affairs of the Sanitary Commission, Rose was free to leave the country. He sailed from New York on August 2 and arrived in London in time to meet with the delegates to the 17th International Congress of Medicine at a dinner given by Sir Thomas Barlow, personal physician to King George V and president of the Congress. Among the some 150 physicians from all over the Empire who heard Rose that evening was F. M. Sandwith, a former co-worker with Looss in Egypt on the experiments that showed the life history of the hookworm. Two nights later, on Wednesday, August 12, Page gave a dinner in Rose's honor at the Marlborough Club. In attendance were several important physicians in both the colonial service and the London medical hierarchy as well as two highly placed figures in the Foreign Office — Lewis Harcourt, Secretary of State for the Colonies, and Lord Crewe, Secretary of State for India. Rose's formal remarks included a review of the Sanitary Commission's activities, illustrated with 70 lantern slides, and an offer on behalf of his colleagues on the International Health Commission to assist the British in moving against hookworm disease in the countries of the Empire. He was surprised to find his audience already highly knowledgeable on the subject of hookworm infection in the tropics and receptive to an offer of assistance to work toward its eradication. Harcourt, speaking on behalf of the Colonial Office, predicted that they would all look back on the evening "as the beginning of a new day in the administration of our colonial affairs, and of a better civilization for all countries in the tropics."[26] Sandwith congratulated Rose for making more headway "in one evening than we have been able to . . . at all."[27] Unlike the physicians in the colonial service, however, Rose came bearing, not seeking, gifts. Before he returned to New York, Rose had secured accreditation in all Britain's colonies, and he and his hosts had worked out a program by which the International Health Commission would first concentrate its efforts in the British West Indies, with Egypt, Ceylon, and Malaya to follow, leaving the larger and more complex Indian subcontinent until the American hookworm doctors had amassed some practical experience. Rose agreed to visit in the near future each country in which work was contemplated. After a brief round of sightseeing (he found England beautiful, "a domesticated land" — as well he might, after his success in London), he sailed for New York, sixteen days after his arrival.[28]

Rose was back in the United States for about a month before he embarked on a tour of the British possessions in the Caribbean basin. After attending back-to-back meetings of the Sanitary Commission's and the International Health Commission's executive committees on the morning of October 4, he set sail in the afternoon for Barbados, in the company, as it happened, of Theodore Roosevelt, off to the jungles of Brazil in search of a better navel orange. Rose spent the next two months with British colonial administrators and physicians inspecting local conditions on Barbados, Trinidad, British Guiana, Grenada, St. Vincent, St. Lucia, and Antigua. He found hookworm disease prevalent in six of the seven colonies he visited, and made tentative arrangements for beginning the work. In December 1913, he was back in the United States again, but only long enough to prepare the Sanitary Commission's fourth annual report, attend the January annual meetings, and put in motion plans to send International Health Commission doctors to the West Indies. On March 9, 1914, less than a year after the incorporation of the Rockefeller Foundation, an agent of the International Health Commision, Hector H. Howard, arrived in British Guiana. A veteran of the hookworm campaign in Mississippi, Howard had also been Bass' old partner in the Columbia practice.[29]

By the time Howard reached Georgetown, Rose was already off again, this time on the first leg of a five-month trip around the world. In London he was joined by Sandwith ("strong in practical judgment," according to Rose). Their first stop was in Egypt, where Lord Kitchener, the governor-general, agreed to match with government funds Rose's offer of £6,000 to initiate a hookworm program in the Nile Valley. Hobnobbing with Kitchener, soon to become the recruiting poster symbol of indomitable Britain, was the sort of thing that had become part of a day's work for Rose. The repressed Southerner in him, however, found nothing commonplace (according to an entry in his journal) about a chance encounter at the Sphinx with the daughter of Robert E. Lee.[30]

Ceylon followed Egypt. Here Rose left Sandwith, his Passepartout for the first half of the journey, before continuing alone to Panay, Singapore, and Manila. Victor G. Heiser, head of the U.S. Public Health Service in the Philippines at the time of Rose's visit but soon to join the International Health Commission, led him to believe that the American colonial officials would also co-operate fully with the representatives of the Rockefeller Founda-tion. Rose arrived back in the United States shortly before the outbreak of the First World War. He had spent eight of the pre-ceding twelve months abroad, and he had every reason to be ela-ted about the way things had developed. From all indications, it appeared likely that hookworm disease would prove to be, as he had prophesied and as Gates had foreseen, the "entering wedge" for the Rockefeller Foundation around the world.[31]

It remained for someone to administer the *coup de grâce* to the Sanitary Commission. Since Gates had been the one who had se-cretly and unilaterally decided its fate, he was the fitting person to play the executioner. After Rose had left the country on his trip around the world, Gates acted swiftly to bring the work in the South to a close. But he bungled his thankless assignment badly and threw a pall of confusion, bitterness, and disillusion-ment over the last months of the Sanitary Commission's ex-istence.

In his few weeks in Washington between his various trips abroad, Rose had discussed with Ferrell, his assistant, tentative plans for merging the work of the Sanitary Commission smoothly and gradually into the new programs of the International Health Commission. But apparently he did not bring his ideas to the at-tention of his fellow Commissioners on the Sanitary Commission at either the annual meeting in January 1914 or the meeting of the executive committee a few days later. Ferrell's desk book con-tains an entry, dated January 19, 1914, reminding him to remind Rose to "ascertain [the] temper of the Commission on aiding in getting a thorough trial for the whole-time community physician idea,"[32] but the minutes of the subsequent meeting do not contain any reference to a discussion of this or any of the more general as-pects of transition. Perhaps Rose chose not to put the matter squarely on the table once he had been satisfied, early in the meet-ing, that a couple of small straws in the wind (such as the exten-sion beyond the end of 1914 of the terms of office for Stiles and four other Commissioners) seemed to indicate that the Sanitary Commission was not fated for an abrupt liquidation. Two days before he sailed for London on the first leg of his five-month voy-age, Rose prepared a memorandum for Ferrell in which he set forth guidelines for carrying on the work in the South during his absence. Nothing in his last-minute instructions suggested that he foresaw the need for making plans to bring the Sanitary Commission's activities to a close in the immediate future. "The time has come," he wrote, "for intensive community work . . . Among the conditions favoring success in such communities are the following: a. A whole-time county health officer for the county in which the community is located. b. The community to be typically rural. c. A reasonably heavy infection. d. Promise of securing cooperation of the people. e. A school with a live teacher that will give active cooperation."[33] These do not sound like the words of a man resigned to abandoning the Southern campaign. At another place in the memorandum Rose argued: "We ought to put forth every effort in the next two or three years to bring about definite results in the way of improved sanitation."[34]

Shortly after Rose's departure, Ferrell was summoned to New York for a meeting of the International Health Commission's (not the Sanitary Commission's) executive committee. In attendance were the younger Rockefeller, Gates, Greene, Murphy, and Flexner. Gates moved that the Sanitary Commission's activities be terminated at the end of the year and instructed Ferrell, in Rose's absence, to draft and submit proposals toward that end. Ferrell later recalled arguing that since Rose had already formulated plans to integrate the remaining goals of the Sanitary Commission into the new programs of the International Health Commission, it would perhaps be better to suspend action on Gates's motions until after Rose's return. Gates replied that he had been the one who was responsible for the creation of the Sanitary Commission in the first place and that Rockefeller's gift had carried the stipulation that the campaign was to last only five years. On his return to Washington, Ferrell sent word to the state health officers, and through them to the field workers and other employees, that the Sanitary Commission would very likely be going out of business at the end of the year. He asked each state director to forward as quickly as possible suggestions for rounding out the work in his state.[35]

Gates had been quite correct in observing that the Sanitary Commission had been originally created for five years. He also intimated privately that in his opinion the South could ill afford to support both the ongoing public schools programs of the General Education Board and a protracted campaign to upgrade its public health facilities. It was his belief that in the General Education Board's efforts to improve Southern agriculture and public schooling lay the shortest and safest route to a greater regional prosperity which in turn would lead to a more favorable economic environment for public health work. He reiterated as well his belief that the Sanitary Commission had already adequately demonstrated to the people of the South what they needed to do, but that it was now their responsibility to see that it got done. He failed to include among his reasons for scrapping the Sanitary Commission (although there are several strong indications that it was preying on his mind at the time) the fact that the reputation of the Rockefellers had recently sunk so low following clashes between National Guardsmen and striking coal miners in Colorado that no American program which bore their name – philanthropic or otherwise, ongoing or new – could hope to achieve or retain popular support.

In September 1913, ten thousand Colorado miners had walked off the job in protest against conditions in the mines and mining villages and against the producers' refusal to recognize the United Mine Workers as a bargaining agent. Violence, sometimes approaching the level of guerrilla warfare, broke out almost immediately and continued throughout the winter and early spring of 1914. The largest of the producers, a major power in Colorado politics and the leader in the movement to resist the strikers' demands, was the Colorado Fuel and Iron Company. The Rockefellers owned 40 percent of the common and preferred stock in Colorado Fuel and Iron and over 43 percent of its bonds. Gates's uncle, L. M. Bowers, was the chairman of its board of directors. The Rockefellers' interest and influence in the company was so generally known that on September 15, 1913, with the walkout looming, the chief negotiator from the Labor Department approached Rockefeller, Jr. with a request – which was turned aside – to intercede in the interest of a peaceful compromise. Several times in the next seven months, both Rockefeller, Jr. and Gates encouraged Bowers to stand firm against the miners. There is evidence to suggest that Bowers, with the younger Rockefeller's enthusiastic approval, brought intense pressure to bear on Elias M. Ammons, "our little cowboy governor," in Bowers' words, to use the National Guard prejudicially to protect strikebreakers and to intimidate strikers. In testimony before a subcommittee of the House Committee on Mines and Mining, the younger Rockefeller endorsed Bowers' intransigence and upheld the principle of the open shop, even at the risk of open warfare between the company and its disaffected employees.

Finally, on the morning of April 20, 1914, a company of skittish state militia occupying positions on a hill overlooking a ramshackle tent city in Ludlow, Colorado, opened fire on the striking miners and their families. Forty people died in the exchange of gunfire; many more were wounded; and when the smoke cleared, the Ludlow survivors discovered the bodies of two women and eleven children, dead of suffocation in a cellar where they had taken refuge from their burning tent. In the immediate aftermath of the Ludlow killings, other striking miners went on a rampage, seizing towns and destroying company offices across the state. Only a detachment of federal troops, rushed to the scene on orders from President Wilson, could end the fighting and restore a semblance of calm.[36]

The public outcry following the bloody events in Colorado was not limited to a few radicals and labor agitators. Whatever else might be said about the Rockefeller's and Gates's involvement in the Ludlow fiasco,[37] everyone agreed that they now had a full-blown public relations problem on their hands. The younger Rockefeller immediately put aside a long-standing family aversion to the mechanics of self-promotion by hiring Ivy Lee, a specialist in rehabilitating the reputations of American business-men, "to make our position clear."[38] The rest of the trustees of the Rockefeller Foundation also took immediate steps to limit the damage to their patrons' public images in whatever ways they could. Jerome Greene and President Charles W. Eliot of Harvard, a Foundation trustee and Greene's former employer, invited the Canadian industrial relations expert, W. L. Mackenzie King, to come to New York ostensibly to discuss a Foundation project, in fact to persuade him to go to work for the Rockefellers. Foundation grants were hastily awarded to Colorado College (whose president subsequently provided Lee with good, anti-union quotations for inclusion in a Rockefeller propaganda bulletin), the University of Denver (whose dean of liberal arts did likewise), and the Colorado Committee on Unemployment.[39]

Perhaps it was only natural for the younger Rockefeller to defend himself with whatever means were at hand in his time of need. But when those means included a gigantic foundation pledged to serve "the well-being of mankind," his critics, their numbers swollen after Ludlow, also quite naturally pointed to what they saw as the hypocrisy at the very heart of this allegedly dispassionate benevolent institution. Frank Walsh, the Chairman of the U.S. Commission on Industrial Relations which conducted widely publicized hearings into the coal-field disturbances and Rockefeller's culpability in them,[40] warned that the fledgling Foundation was dangerous as well as hypocritical. The historian James Weinstein found an unpublished essay of Walsh's entitled

"The Great Foundations," which argues that not even the pure scientific research projects were to be commended. Weinstein has summarized Walsh's argument:

[Walsh] challenged "the wisdom of giving public sanction and approval to the spending of a huge fortune through such philanthropies" and viewed such "philanthropic trusts" as a "menace to the welfare of society." The possession of such enormous fortunes meant "arbitrary power over the lives and destinies of other men," Walsh wrote, adding that "the forms of political democracy avail nothing when the lives of the many are controlled by the few who wield arbitrary economic power." Walsh insisted that "even in the power to do good, no one man, or group of men, should hold a monopoly." The setting up of scientific or social work foundations, Walsh warned, must lead to a condition of "loyalty and subserviency"to men of wealth and their "interests from the whole profession of scientists, social workers, and economists." Already there were "thousands of men in these professions receiving subsidies, either directly or indirectly, from the Rockefeller Estate." These men were in a position where to "take any step toward effective economic, social and industrial reform" would bring them "directly counter to the interests of their benefactor." No sensible man can believe, Walsh insisted, "that research workers, publicists and teachers can be subsidized with money obtained from the exploitation of workers without being profoundly influenced in their points of view and in the energy and enthusiasm with which they might otherwise attack economic abuses."[41]

Attenuated echoes of such criticism—this time with specific reference to the work of the Sanitary Commission—rippled the surface of Charles V. Chapin's widely discussed survey of state boards of health. The dean of American municipal public health officers, Chapin of Providence had been commissioned by the American Medical Association in the fall of 1913 to make a comprehensive comparative study of the activities, staffs, budgets, and facilities of the various state boards of health. Although his final report did not appear until 1915, his general conclusions were the subject of much heated discussion among public health workers in the two years before his results were published. Chapin credited the Sanitary Commission with an awakening of interest in public health in the eleven Southern states it had entered, and noted that "the Commission brought health to thousands, demonstrated an important preventable disease, showed how its cause could be removed and brought about a marked sanitary improvement in countless dwellings and schools."[42] Like Walsh, however, Chapin worried about the potential for abuse inherent in the relationship between benefactor and beneficiary. "It appears to an outsider," he wrote, "that while the

Commission nominally acts through the state health department it really carries on its work as an independent organization. Indeed it could scarcely be otherwise. It is difficult for an employee to serve two masters." The built-in dangers in the structure of control developed by the Sanitary Commission went a long way, in Chapin's opinion, toward offsetting its benefits. "There are many who feel that it is dangerous to have outside agencies initiate and direct the activities of state and municipal officials. There is scarcely a health officer who has not had help from one private organization or another. Yet there is probably not a health officer who is not in constant fear that some group of over-enthusiastic, and perhaps ill-advised, reformers may not, by outside pressure, bring about a one-sided diversion of the funds of his department, perhaps to lines of work of problematical value."[43] Walsh would have added, "and with hidden motives."

Walsh's warnings, Chapin's reservations, the spontaneous outpouring of hatred toward the Rockefellers in the wake of the Ludlow killings, the turmoil in the New York offices—all these factors, perhaps more than the ones enumerated by Gates, made the prospect of overseas work among submissive colonials increasingly more attractive.

Intimations that the Sanitary Commission's days were numbered touched off a predictable furor among its rank and file. Part of their incredulity no doubt stemmed from a feeling of betrayal; after all, Ferrell himself had written less than a year earlier, "I see no occasion for a man who is making good in the work to feel uneasy about its duration."[44] Rose returned from his trip around the world to find the morale among his field workers—so good when he had embarked five months earlier—now destroyed. Freeman wrote from Virginia, "My sensations during the last few days have been very much akin to those of a man who painstakingly and carefully builds a house of cards and then in an instant sees the whole thing fall to the ground ... I feel depressed with the sense of failure, that we have failed to make our work so necessary as to insure its perpetuation, and that is the feeling that dominates the present situation."[45] Rose felt betrayed himself. Gates had acted on his own, without taking Rose into his confidence, and had left him to deal with the unpleasant consequences of a decision Rose had not helped to make and did not endorse. He vented his frustration in a reply to Freeman's letter. "I find it difficult to say more than that I agree with your point of view," he wrote. "This is a fine piece of sanitary machinery; it has done a good bit of work ... I agree with you that the disorganization of this machine represents a serious loss."[46] Dinsmore wrote from Alabama that he could no longer in good conscience go through with plans to open intensive community work in his state. Leathers in Mississippi worried about the permanency of the results if the campaign were halted so precipitately. From Arkansas the state health officer wrote that without the presence of the Sanitary Commission, his public health bill pending in the state legislature would be in serious trouble. McCormack in Kentucky was reluctant to pass the shutdown announcement along to his field workers: "As soon as this resolution is transmitted, we will lose all three of our inspectors, as, of course, it will take the heart out of our work and they will be anxious to make their permanent plans for the future."[47]

So great was Rose's frustration that he gave serious thought to the possibility of resigning both his posts with the Rockefeller philanthropies. Jerome Greene found him "deeply grieved and disappointed."[48] In vain he argued that it made about as little sense to shut down the Sanitary Commission in 1914 as it would have a year earlier; at neither point had any of the original objectives been truly achieved. Gates would not be dissuaded, but he did try to mollify Rose. "To start a philanthropy like the Hookworm work in the South is difficult," he wrote. "To conduct it to a conspicuous success is more difficult. But to stop it at the right moment, when all that is *true* success has been achieved, *that* is the most difficult of all – an achievement most rare and given only to the choicest and most rigorous spirits . . . The damage in stopping the work, *whatever* that be to workers or *others*, is as nothing to the damage inflicted upon society by continuing a work for it with foreign means *after a reasonable local enlightenment has created the local responsibility for self help* and the means of self help exist. For that is to *sap the foundations of character and social life itself*."[49] Several men on the Sanitary Commission, including the younger Rockefeller and Stiles, and several others on the International Health Commission, Eliot and Greene among them, were prepared to take Rose's side if he decided to force the issue with Gates. But Rose elected to back down and let Gates have his way uncontested. Perhaps it was in part because Rose, as Fosdick recalled, "was a mouse-like man, self-effacing,"[50] and reluctant to lock horns with the more tempestuous Gates. More likely he knew that resistance was futile since Gates had already won over the elder Rockefeller to his point of view. In a typed, six-page letter to his employer, Gates had carefully and persuasively set out his reasons for discontinuing the Sanitary Commission:

Dr. Rose has done his work well. His plans were well conceived, his methods effective, the results have been comprehensive and decisive. Against universal incredulity, he has secured universal recognition of the existence, the wide distribution, and, in places, the destructiveness of the disease. He has disclosed its cause, its method of propagation, its symptoms, its treatment and cure, its prevention . . . He has cured more than half a million, has traversed the most heavily infected districts with traveling hospitals, has evoked immense popular interest, called forth no inconsiderable public aid, and practically banished the disease as epidemic from the regions for the most part where it has been found to be seriously destructive. He has awakened the Boards of Health in all the states to the existence and distribution of the infection in their several states, has secured for them special legislative appropriations, has shown them models of effective state organization and county and local canvass. He has trained them in the use of all this machinery by employing them as his own agents. He has not only enlisted county aid, but with the greatest unanimity, the whole body of local physicians in every county of every state. No disease is better known, more easily recognized or more promptly cured by the average southern physician. The work we undertook to do has been done within the time fixed, done within . . . the sum we thought necessary, and very much more has been done than we then planned or thought possible. Hookworm disease has not only been recognized, bounded and limited, it has been reduced to one of the minor infections of the south, perhaps the most easily and universally recognized and cured of all. This *now*. More than this, a most admirably adapted and equipped state machine has been set up in each state, ready at hand, for the local authorities to employ whenever further work is thought of sufficient importance to justify public funds . . . Needless further aid from us is damaging rather than necessary or helpful. So I say to Dr. Rose, "well done, good and faithful servant. Thou has been faithful over a few things, we will make thee ruler over many things; henceforth, thy field is the world."[51]

Rose was able to persuade Gates to permit the work in some states to continue for six months into 1915. Gates insisted, however, that it be done under the auspices of the International Health Commission. Rose's acceptance of this compromise signaled the end of his resistance. The way was now prepared for the formal announcement of the Sanitary Commission's termination. On August 12, 1914, the elder Rockefeller sent a letter to the members of the Commission. It was undoubtedly written by Gates.

My pledge of October 26, 1909, for the support of your work in the southern states was made for a period of five years, which period may be interpreted as coming to an end not later than December 31, 1914. I understand that in planning your budget covering work in progress during the current year, you are making no commitments beyond that date. The work thus far accomplished would seem to have brought about in all of the southern states a very general knowledge on the part of physicians, health authorities and the public regarding the prevalence of hookworm disease and the methods of treating and may thus be deemed to have been accomplished. Realizing, however, that there may be places in which a consistent plan of work would require the continuation of your efforts for a time, I request that the necessity for such continuation be referred by you, with appropriate recommendations thereon, to The Rockefeller Foundation, which is in a position, by reason of its permanent character and endowment, to continue, extend or modify the work, if it shall so elect, as in its judgment may from time to time be expedient. It is my desire that all property acquired by your commission, including records, files, reports, medical supplies, furniture and equipment, be transferred and delivered to The Rockefeller Foundation on or before December 31, 1914.

In thus arranging for the termination of your effective and beneficient labors, which have earned the just gratitude of our southern people, I wish to thank you one and all for the great service which you have rendered.[52]

Rose drew up a plan whereby the work would be brought to a close in six states (Virginia, South Carolina, Mississippi, Louisiana, Arkansas, and Kentucky) on December 31, 1914. The International Health Commission would fund anti-hookworm programs in North Carolina and Alabama through March 31, 1915, and in Texas, Tennessee, and Georgia through June 30, 1915. No dispensary work remained to be accomplished in North Carolina, but Rose thought it wise to extend eradication experiments in several communities there, especially since the North Carolina State Board of Health had agreed to pay one-half of the expenses. Alabama, Texas, Tennessee, and Georgia all had counties with a high incidence of hookworm infection in which no dispensary work had as yet been undertaken. Tennessee's and Georgia's field forces were to be augmented by one and five physicians, respectively. The additional sanitary inspectors and microscopists would move over from states in which all Sanitary Commission work had been concluded.[53]

McCormack had reason to worry about the future of his Kentucky field workers. None of them was asked to go to work for the International Health Commission. In fact, only seven doctors from two states — out of 109 in eleven states on the Sanitary Commission staff in 1914 — were taken into the new organization. One of the seven, Merrill E. Champion, a recent graduate of the Harvard medical school, had been placed on the Sanitary Commission's staff in 1914 expressly for the purpose of gaining experience in intensive community work before moving over to the International Health Commission. One state director, M. H. Boerner of Texas, declined an invitation to stay on, and one former field worker, Benjamin Washburn, joined the International Health Commission after an interlude as a North Carolina county health officer. Allen Freeman continued in public health work with the Virginia State Department of Health, and with his assistance, three members of his field staff were able to find work of one sort or another in the field of public health. Leathers in Mississippi was appointed State Health Officer after the dissolution of the Sanitary Commission. The vast majority of Sanitary Commission employees, however, were left to fend for themselves. Even if one includes Washburn in the tally, the fact remains that only seven percent of the Sanitary Commission's staff of full-time physicians found work with the International Health Commission. Howard and Rowan came from Leathers' Mississippi corps; from North Carolina, Ferrell brought Jacocks, Champion, Covington, Kibler, and later, Washburn. Apparently, now that it was no longer necessary to consider Southern sensibilities when choosing personnel, Rose and his assistants no longer felt compelled to recruit recent graduates of Southern medical schools but could hire instead alumni of the better medical schools of the Northeast.[54]

The man who was widely heralded as the "discoverer" of hookworm disease in the United States, who had preached its dangers longer than anyone else, knew more about it than any other scientist or medical man alive, and first called it to the attention of Rockefeller's advisers, was not invited to join the International Health Commission. Far too important a figure to settle for a job as an ordinary overseas field worker, Charles Wardell Stiles had proved too much the maverick to be asked to serve on its executive staff. In recent years, he had found himself in vociferous opposition to a pet project or scheme of at least three of the men who might have put forward his name for consideration. He had first challenged the value of Rose's beloved dispensary program, then quarreled heatedly with Ferrell over an acceptable privy model, and finally decried Gates's decision to shut down the Sanitary Commission. Moreover, his irascibility was not reserved for his colleagues on the Sanitary Commission but spilled over into his relationships with subordinates. Between 1912 and the end of 1914, for example, he went through five personal secretaries. Despite his long and distinguished career in government service,

Stiles was just not a good company man. Whatever there was about him that made him the perfect John the Baptist of the anti-hookworm work also made it impossible for Stiles to switch easily into the role of an apostle in Rockefeller's public health bureaucracy created specifically to combat "his" disease.

His refusal to go gently only served to confirm those who were dismissing him in the soundness of their decision. His rage at being left behind was both heartfelt and curiously misdirected. Gates was unassailable, and at any rate his hand in the decision was well concealed. Rose had been out of the country when the word went out from Washington that the Sanitary Commission's days were numbered. Ferrell was left alone to bear the brunt of Stiles's wrath. From Stiles's point of view, he made a good target. Stiles had already begun to resent him several years earlier when Ferrell, in his capacity as the North Carolina state director, had crossed Stiles repeatedly in an attempt to bring the scientific secretary's independent work in Wilmington into line with the statewide program. Stiles's suspicions had grown when Ferrell was summoned to Washington in 1913 to become Rose's assistant, a move that Stiles viewed as a tacit reduction of his own influence as the sole scientific voice on the Sanitary Commission's executive committee. Suspicions blossomed into open antagonism over the issue of safe versus economical privies. The shutdown order thus seemed to Stiles to represent the final act in a successful coup that Ferrell had been planning for months. At a hastily called meeting of the state directors in Richmond, held after the unofficial termination inquiry had been circulated but before Rose's return, Stiles lashed out at Ferrell, accusing him of falsifying the North Carolina results during his tenure as state director in order to curry favor with Rose and of plotting the Sanitary Commission's demise to further his own ambition to be a director of the new International Health Commission. Stiles distributed a bill of particulars against Ferrell among his associates on the Commission and among the state directors, most of whom were already disgruntled, many of whom claimed never to have been informed of the five-year proviso. Hidden in the intemperate *ad hominem* attack on Ferrell was Stiles's impassioned plea to stay the execution of the Sanitary Commission. The full measure of his eclipse is to be found in the casual manner with which Stiles's colleagues dismissed his final *cri de coeur*. Gates urged Ferrell to brush it off; Greene and Flexner labeled it the ill-considered outburst of a frustrated man. In a last petulant gesture six months later, Stiles delayed for a few weeks the publication of the Sanitary Commission's fifth and final annual report by withholding the scientific secretary's section.[55]

The work of the Sanitary Commission may have been brought to a close on a messy, acrimonious note, but its sour demise in no way diminished Gates's enthusiasm for the prospective endeavors of the International Health Commision. Rose's impressive diplomatic successes in London and around the world only seemed to validate Gates's long-standing conviction that medicine and public health offered irreproachable opportunities for philanthropy. Disease was a problem so endemic and so universally recognized that it was almost a part of the very definition of the human condition. "Disease," wrote Gates, "is the supreme ill of human life, and it is the main source of almost all other human ills, poverty, crime, ignorance, vice, inefficiency, hereditary taint, and many other evils."[56] Other reformers and philanthropists busied themselves treating the symptoms of this more deep-seated disorder; or, as Gates believed, "the great mass of charities of the world concern themselves directly or indirectly with relieving or mitigating such evils and miseries of society as are due mainly to disease."[57] Moreover, reformers and philanthropists who restricted their efforts to the social, political, or economic consequences of disease wasted too much effort in disagreements among themselves. One reformer's panacea was another's ideological poison. Gates, who felt strongly that "the evils of society are not fundamentally economic but are physical and moral,"[58] lamented the fact that most reformers of this sort bickered over the best means of achieving what he considered to be superficial objectives. The medical researcher or public health doctor stood well above the fray, *sans peur et sans reproche*. His work not only plunged more deeply toward the source of all human suffering but also, in Gates's view, was immune to criticism regarding ends and means. Gates was to rue the day, only a few years later, when the Rockefeller Foundation expanded the scope of its activities, against his advice, to include problems of a social nature, but for the time being, as long as he exercised control over policy, its programs would be limited to medicine and public health.

Gates was emphatic on this point, but the question still remains, what was there specifically about hookworm disease that appealed so much to him? Why did he choose it, long before the results of the Sanitary Commission were in, to serve as the Rockefeller Foundation's entering wedge? From a strictly medical point of view, hookworm disease proved both a fortunate and fortuitous choice. John Ferrell, while he was still the state director of the North Carolina hookworm campaign, summarized the advantages that an anti-hookworm program offered over a comparable effort against any of the other diseases—oftentimes more deadly, invariably more spectacular—confronting the public health worker. Ferrell began by reasserting what had come to be a commonplace among public health officials—that their work was as much educational as medical. What disease, he asked, "afforded the best opportunity for the eternal demonstration"? Ferrell then ticked off, one by one, the major Southern public health threats: diptheria, malaria, typhoid fever, tuberculosis; each certainly took its grim annual toll, but none lent itself well to the educational goals of Southern sanitarians. Diptheria struck sporadically; malaria was seasonal; typhoid fever, incurable; and tuberculosis, intractable.

Hookworm disease has none of these disadvantages. It is the most prevalent disease we have and is found in every county of the State. Its chronic nature renders it available for demonstrative purposes every day of the year in every community of the State. It is the only one of the common diseases in the State which has a causative agent discernible to the naked eye. It is both preventable and curable by methods the simplicity of which appeals to everyone. The results following treatment are so prompt and emphatic that they have been aptly compared with the miracles of the New Testament.[59]

Ferrell applauded the remarkable prescience that had led the Rockefeller group to limit its first public health venture to this one disease. Unforeseen benefits would surely accrue from that decision. "In a long and profitable experience with petroleum," Ferrell added, Rockefeller "had learned that the byproducts of his industry rival in importance the refined oil."[60]

Perhaps so. Clearly from Ferrell's point of view at least, hookworm disease was the answer to a sanitarian's prayer. But Gates and his associates who organized and directed the work of the Sanitary Commission out of the Rockefeller offices were neither physicians nor public health workers. Only Stiles, an outsider, had any experience before 1909 in directing public health programs. That professionals in the field approved their choice long after the fact was no doubt reassuring, but it hardly explains the reasons behind the choice in the first place.

Others since Ferrell have offered competing explanations. In his study of the early Rockefeller medical philanthropies, including the Sanitary Commission, E. Richard Brown has argued that Gates acted consistently from within his entrepreneurial class perspective, in the interests of the United States dominant industrial elite whose values and assumptions he shared.[61] Early in his tenure with the Rockefellers, Gates realized that the emerging scientific medicine could be employed with telling effect by America's capitalists *qua* philanthropists in their struggle to consolidate and strengthen their grip on society. Preventive medicine, with its recurring metaphors equating a healthy body to a smoothly functioning machine, would ensure the increased efficiency of the working class, thus binding its defective (and disaffected) components more closely to the industrial process. Each of the Rockefeller medical programs, Brown concludes, "can be traced to Gates's . . . broader concern for the permanent economic and social viability of capitalist society."[62] The Sanitary Commission, then, was just one of several institutional embodiments of this capitalist world view. Brown contends that "Whatever genuine pride the Rockefellers and Gates felt in relieving the suffering of thousands of Southerners, their primary incentive was clearly the increased productivity of workers freed of the endemic parasite."[63] As evidence he cites a letter from Gates to the elder Rockefeller on the inefficiency of the hookworm-ridden Southern cotton mill operatives.

In his doctoral dissertation, Howard S. Berliner has drawn out a very similar argument to greater length. He traces Gates's decision to declare global war on hookworm disease to two sources: a secularized missionary impulse and a misapplication of the germ theory of disease. Other investigators before Berliner – Merle Curti and Ernest R. May prominent among them – uncovered a definite link between nineteenth-century American overseas missionary activity and both American philanthropy abroad and American foreign policy in the twentieth century.[64] Gates himself acknowledged the philanthropist's (as well as the businessman's and the consumer's) debt to the path-breaking work of the missionaries. There can be little doubt that both Gates and Rockefeller, deeply religious men with a record of support for missions at home and abroad, had the missionary example uppermost in their minds when they set up the International Health Commission. The younger Rockefeller was himself a devout Baptist and a Sunday school teacher. Jerome Greene's great-grandfather had helped to found the American Board of Commissioners for Foreign Missions; his grandfather had served as one of its officers; his parents had been among its first representatives to Japan (where Greene was born); and his father had assisted in the first Japanese translation of the Bible. The composition of both the

Rockefeller Foundation's original board of trustees and the leadership of the International Health Commission definitely reflected the nineteenth-century American missionary experience. In addition, two other early programs of the Foundation bear a missionary stamp. The China Medical Board, organized in February 1914, came into being largely on the basis of testimony from Christian medical missionaries to that most popular of all heathen lands. In April 1914, the trustees of the Foundation approved a petition presented by John R. Mott of the Y.M.C.A. on behalf of a group of independent missionary boards soliciting Rockefeller funds to outfit and maintain a central office in New York out of which foreign missionary activity might be coordinated.[65]

Berliner's other contention – that Gates chose hookworm disease because it accorded well with his curious understanding of the germ theory of disease – is not as readily apparent as his first and requires closer scrutiny. He has suggested that Gates, like Rockefeller a successful capitalist with a stake in an unfettered economic system and a class interest in seeing it strengthened and expanded, seized upon the germ theory of disease and used it to further his own conservative social, political, and economic ends. Historians have long been aware of the unscientific purposes to which scientific theories have been put. Richard Hofstadter and others have claimed that apologists for laissez-faire capitalism modified Darwin's theory of natural selection to justify their social views, and Charles C. Gillispie has suggested that English mineowners in the Regency Period utilized the geological discoveries of their day to prove to their miners that stratification – be it among rock formations below ground or social classes above – was indeed God's way.[66] Thus Berliner: "The mechanical and reductionist understanding of disease, fostered by the germ theory, lent itself well to the industrial mentality of the time, which lent further credibility to the theory in the eyes of philanthropically inclined entrepreneurs."[67] The hookworm, as everyone knew, was the "germ of laziness." By inaugurating a campaign to eradicate hookworm disease, Gates hoped, in Berliner's opinion, to draw attention away from the inequities inherent in the American economic system, such as dietary deficiencies brought about by marginal incomes, that contributed to the proliferation of disease in the first place. "By focusing the attack on the hookworm, as the Rockefeller Sanitary Commission did, the role of diet, clearly related to income, was ignored."[68] Before Gates could commit Rockefeller's money to a program to combat hookworm disease he had first, in Berliner's view, to exaggerate its dangers.

While it is certainly true that Page, at least, did magnify the hookworm's impact on man's health and man's institutions, there is no evidence to suggest that Gates did. American and European parasitologists in 1909 believed that the presence of hookworms in the intestines above a certain number (the number varied) posed a definite threat to human health. Gates made his decisions based on information available to him at the time. No reports to the effect that hookworms were harmless enough if their host's diet was iron-rich existed in the medical literature in 1909.[69] Opposition to the anti-hookworm work of the Sanitary Commission almost always took the form of skepticism over the alleged prevalence, not the virulence, of the disease. Once the results of the early state infection surveys were made known, diehard critics like Candler were forced to refocus their attack on Rockefeller's involvement in the work, for they could no longer dismiss out of hand the need to do something about the hookworm.

Leaving aside the question of economic influences on Gates's mentality, Berliner's identification of the connection between Gates's fascination with the germ theory of disease (picked up from reading Osler) and his later decision to target hookworm disease points toward a fuller explanation of Gates's motives. Gates himself acknowledged the importance of Osler to the development of his ideas on medicine and disease. In his autobiography, he treats his introduction to the famous textbook almost as an epiphanal moment in his life. It seems therefore most likely, knowing what we do about Gates, that Osler's description of the germ theory struck in him a much deeper chord than the one Berliner points out. Briefly put, the germ theory of disease bore a remarkable resemblance to the old evangelical notion of sin which had been drummed into Gates as a child and later as a seminarian.

If proponents of the germ theory believed that man was subject to assault from all sides by microorganisms capable of undermining his health, pietists believed that he was a weak creature in another sense, vulnerable to a host of specifically enumerated temptations. If the scientists and physicians who read Pasteur and Koch tended to ignore the importance of the environment as a contributing factor in the generation and proliferation of disease, the evangelists who followed Wesley first and later Finney tended to stress the importance of the individual's direct relationship with God, and not his allegiance to the wider community of

Christians. If advocates of the germ theory viewed a specific disease as an aggregate of afflicted persons, pietists regarded a specific social problem, such as slavery, as the effect on society of countless individual sinners. If it is true that subscribers to the germ theory reduced disease to a simple matter of identifying and treating the bacteriological agent, it is equally true that evangelical Christians attacked a social evil by attempting first to identify the sin that caused it and then to cleanse each sinner who helped perpetuate it. Etiology – the concept, if not the word itself – played as important a part in the pietist's definition of the relationship between sin and social health as it did in the bacteriologist's theory regarding the link between germs and disease.[70]

Gates and Rockefeller were certainly steeped in the habits of mind and the traditions of evangelical religion. Both had acquired their pietistic instincts in the backwoods, far from those centers of American industry in existence in the mid-nineteenth century, long before either became a successful capitalist entrepreneur. Both had come lately to their class perspectives, but they had been born and brought up in the bosom of evangelical Protestantism.

To someone like Gates with an evangelical cast of mind, regardless of how far he thought he might have come from his days as a Baptist, hookworm disease – more than any other "germ"-related human ailment – could easily have become an unconscious cognate of sin itself.[71] Like sin, it was ubiquitous and quietly persistent, ruining lives but rarely killing its victims outright. Again like sin, it did not strike people from any one station in life; after all, men like Alderman and Houston had recalled the itching feet of their boyhoods. A powerful and pervasive opponent, hookworm disease demanded the unstinting energies of those enlightened few who recognized its dangers. Its cure, however, did not seem to require a complicated or sophisticated environmental approach of the kind eschewed by evangelical Christians. Gates could regard its eradication much as Finney had foreseen the destruction of slavery seventy years earlier: that is, he could bypass politics, the law, economics, and social custom to reach out and touch the life of the individual sufferer (sinner/slave owner). Although the victim of hookworm disease often bore the stigmata of his affliction stamped on his features or inscribed in his behavior, the cure itself was simple and swift. The results were dramatic and virtually instantaneous; the rescued individual was free to move back into the mainstream of society within days, just as the former sinner who had accepted Jesus as his savior could embark on a righteous, productive life as soon as he left the presence of the evangelist. The hookworm treatment—like the mechanics of salvation—required the active and continuing participation of the saved, and like the renunciation of sin, it began quite literally with an exorcism—a regeneration from within. If each hookworm victim could be treated and finally cured, hookworm disease would cease to be a scourge; society would be cleansed. But unless the regenerates were persuaded to adopt a new way of life, the cure would not last. Without vigilance, they would inevitably backslide into disease. The physician, like the evangelist, could exhort the convert to persevere, but in the final analysis it was up to the individual to render witness to his conversion from day to day for the rest of his life. There was nothing peremptory, then, in Gates's decision to liquidate the Sanitary Commission before eradication had been achieved. His reluctance to keep open the flow of Rockefeller money into the South, to dragoon Southerners into building privies until the last hookworm had perished, becomes less mysterious. It was not the evangelist/philanthropist's duty—even if it were in his power—to enforce salvation. Gates's worldwide war on hookworm disease, seen in this light, takes on the features of a secularized crusade, with the dispensary/revival as its mainspring. One can learn what animated it from the top at least as much by studying the career of Billy Sunday as by reading the scientific articles of Charles Wardell Stiles. There was indeed a strong missionary zeal behind the creation of the Rockefeller Foundation—far stronger than is evident at first glance.

To say as much, of course, is not to dismiss as irrelevant reminders of Gates's economic orientation. The two are by no means mutually exclusive. One need not invoke either Weber or his critics in order to acknowledge something more than a coincidental relationship between the protestant ethic and the spirit of capitalism. Why not beg the vexed question of their precise relationship and agree with the historian Paul E. Johnson who, on the basis of his investigation of society and revivals in Rochester during the Jacksonian period, has concluded that "it seems unwise to treat religion and class as separate and competing categories of explanation."[72] Taken together, they can enrich our understanding of Gates, the layman whose approach to medicine was idiosyncratic and emotional and in whose mind, reified under the metamorphic pressure of his felt needs, this odd agglomeration of ideas was put to work in the service of reform.

# Epilogue

Twelve years after the Sanitary Commission closed its doors, the Rockefeller Foundation announced "that hookworm disease has almost disappeared from the United States."[1] The sixty-five-year-old Stiles was taken by surprise. Although he did not believe it for a minute, for the time being he kept his peace. Four years later, shortly before his retirement from the Public Health Service, he made one last tour through the South, visiting schools and examining children. His investigation confirmed his earlier suspicions: in the areas he inspected the rate of infection varied from 26 to 49 percent. In his opinion, the Rockefeller Foundation announcement, "copied very widely in the press," had produced the unfortunate effect "of still further decreasing the school interest in hookworm disease and . . . in inducing many mothers to refuse to accept the diagnosis by physicians and consequently to decline to permit the children to be treated."[2]

To whom at the Rockefeller Foundation could he complain? His closest associates on the Sanitary Commission—Rose, Gates, and Page—were now all dead or retired; Ferrell, in Stiles's estimation, was still untrustworthy. It was to a comparative stranger, Victor Heiser of the International Health Board, that Stiles wrote to express his vigorous disagreement with the Foundation's position that "hooks have become so rare in the U.S.A."[3] Stiles also wrote Rockefeller himself (whom he had never met) urging his old employer to lend his support to an attempt to place the true facts before the health authorities of the United States. When no one in the Rockefeller organization answered him, he took his case against the Foundation to the Washington Biological Society. "I very much regret," he wrote Flexner, "the necessity which has faced me in coming out in public disagreement with The Rockefeller Foundation in regard to the alleged near-eradication of hookworm disease. The publication of the claim by the Foundation was a grave error of judgment and has seriously inhibited hookworm control in the Southern States."[4]

When Flexner also failed to respond to this voice out of the past, Stiles carried his one-sided argument into print. One can imagine his pulse quickening, his indignation starting to mount. This was like the good old days of 1902-1909; then, as now, he had stood alone in opposition to the combined forces of medicine, philanthropy, and public health, most of whom had refused to acknowledge the existence of "his disease." In March 1933, he published an article in *Science* provocatively entitled, "Is It Fair to Say That Hookworm Disease Has Almost Disappeared From the United States?" It *was* fair to say, he acknowledged, that hookworm infection was no longer as virulent and widespread as it had once been – his two-year survey had turned up only fifty dirt-eaters – but there were still enough hookworms in enough Southern schoolchildren to disprove the reckless assertion of the Rockefeller Foundation. "I cannot understand," he wrote, "why the [International Health Board] did not show the . . . strength of character to establish the facts in the case and to admit its mistake."[5]

No one at the Rockefeller Foundation ever saw fit to respond directly to Stiles, much less to admit a mistake. Stiles had raised a good point, however; the statement had been imprudent, if not technically mistaken. Dr. Wilson G. Smillie, author of the disputed assertion, explained to his superior, the director of the International Health Board, that "the real point of difference" between Stiles and himself "relates to the definition of the word *disease*. We make a distinction between hookworm *infection* and hookworm *disease*; he does not. The truth of the matter is, and as everyone familiar with the subject knows, that there are very few individuals left in the United States that are at present suffering with the typical clinical picture of hookworm disease. True hookworm disease, once so familiar in the practice of every physician in the sandy coastal plain of the southern United States has now practically disappeared."[6] Smillie made much of this distinction – "a lawyer's argument," in Raymond Fosdick's opinion[7] – in part because he himself had only recently drawn it. In a 1926 report on the status of hookworm infection in Alabama, he and Dr. Donald L. Augustine noted that in the days of the Sanitary Commission, every case of hookworm infection had been treated as a case of hookworm disease. They concluded that the intensity of infection should concern public health officials more than the extent of its incidence.[8]

Subsequent investigations have tended to uphold Stiles's side of the argument. In the 1930s, public health agencies resurveyed the Southern states for hookworm infection and found a two-thirds decrease since the days of the Sanitary Commission—an important drop, but hardly enough to warrant such a sweeping announcement. Moreover, the same surveys concluded that the geographical distribution of infection in the 1930s was "co-extensive with that of the earlier period."[9] As recently as 1965, Dr. Paul C. Beaver, professor of tropical disease and hygiene at Tulane, found that "hookworm disease was still prevalent in the southeastern United States."[10] On a more personal and much more impressionistic note, the author, while working in a Houston hospital in the mid-1960s, saw the phrase "clay-" or "chalk-eater" on an occasional work-up, usually for patients brought in out of the pine forests of east Texas.

Whatever the merits of either Stiles's or Smillie's argument, the controversy did clarify two things: Stiles could still nettle the Rockefeller Foundation's public health bureaucrats, and the Sanitary Commission had fallen far short of its goal of eradicating hookworm in the Southern states.[11]

In fact, the Sanitary Commission had failed to eradicate hookworm anywhere in the South. Rose had hoped, in the last year of the campaign, that at least one of the intensive community programs, so carefully organized and vigorously pursued, would prove that hookworm could be wiped out in a limited area, if only the right sort of pressure were brought to bear. The twelve selected communities—six in North Carolina, three in Louisiana, two in South Carolina, and one in Virginia—threw themselves into the effort with a commendable civic zeal. Dr. C. L. Pridgen of North Carolina reported to Ferrell that the citizens of Salemburg, in Sampson County, had even come up with a sanitary fight song:

> Brushing, brushing till we're fainting
> Washing, scrubbing, rubbing, painting,
> See we're cleaning, what's the meaning?
> Opportunity!! Model community!![12]

Seaman Knapp's indemnified Texas farmers from the old farm demonstration program would have understood the dynamic tension between pride in being chosen and fear of failure that inspired Salemburg to brush, wash, scrub.

The twelve communities averaged 188 families, 1025 persons, and about 32 square miles of territory. As Rose described it, work in these towns was conducted along two lines: toward the examination of each individual and treatment of the infected ones, and toward renovation of old privies or construction of new ones, as the circumstances dictated. By the end of 1914, only 75 percent of the people in the test communities had been examined, of which 26 percent were found infected; 94 percent of the infected population had been treated; and 29 percent of those, "cured." The actual percentage cured may have been somewhat higher, for in order to ascertain if a patient had been cured, he had to be persistently checked for up to eight weeks, a difficult thing to do even in a labor-intensive program of this nature, conducted in a small town. The results of the Commission's efforts to check soil pollution in these twelve communities indicated that of the 2,257 homes, only about 50 percent had any sort of privy at all when the work began. By the end of 1914, that percentage had risen to 88. When translated into absolute terms, this 76 percent improvement represented the construction of 861 new privies. Brochures touting the accomplishments of the Commission in the twelve test communities were printed and made available as blueprints for similar action in other Southern towns.[13]

The International Health Commission took over and expanded the intensive community program in 1915. Nowhere, however, could it be said that hookworm had been eradicated. The Commission came close in at least one town: in Knott's Island, North Carolina, only "half a dozen old cantankerous people,"[14] who refused to have anything to do with the program, stood between Pridgen and 100 percent participation. In most of the other communities, time ran out for the Commission before its representatives had been give a fair chance to achieve eradication. Rose might console himself in the knowledge that the intensive community programs had brought home to the residents of the participating towns — in a way that the dispensaries had not — the importance of their own roles in maintaining an adequate level of community health. But Rose was frustrated in his desire to see hookworm infection wiped out completely somewhere in the South. The intensive community approach to hookworm control became the central feature of the Internal Health Commission's work overseas, but it came to the Sanitary Commission too late to be of much strategic, or even psychological, value.[15]

In a more technical vein, the Commission also failed to develop an effective, less obnoxious vermifuge to take the place of thymol.

Although both Stiles and Rose knew that many people under-standably refused to take the drug at home because of its often distressing side effects, the scientific secretary was unable to come up with a satisfactory substitute before the Commission went out of business. Thymol was potentially so dangerous that had it been possible, the Commission would have insisted that all doses be administered under careful medical supervision. A hand-ful of people did die as a direct result of thymol dispensed by the Commission. That more did not is either a testimonial to the cau-tion of the Sanitary Commission field workers or an indication that few people actually took the drug at home. The International Health Commission later achieved marginally better results with oil of chenopodium and still later, much better results with car-bon tetrachloride, or one of its variants. Thymol, however, re-mained the standard treatment for hookworm infection for the duration of the Sanitary Commission's work in the South.[16]

Perhaps it should also be counted as a failure of the Commis-sion that its workers could not invent a cheap, satisfactory la-trine. Stiles had his favorite, but few could afford it. Ferrell, with an eye toward expediency, opted for the pit privy, despite evi-dence that it failed to live up to the health standards brought within reach by the technology of the day.

The Sanitary Commission was by no means an unqualified suc-cess. On balance, however, it came remarkably close to achieving its goals, and few would argue that the South was not the better in 1915 for the Commission's presence. With the principles on which the campaign was originally organized and its early struc-ture firmly in mind, it is possible to examine the Commission's achievements in the light of its expressed goals. Before undertak-ing an analysis of this nature, however, one should review the general purpose for the creation of the Commission, from which all the specific goals sprang. Rockefeller's letter of October 26, 1909, stated it clearly for the first time: "The object of the Com-mission shall be to bring about a cooperative movement of the medical profession, public health officials, boards of trade, churches, schools, the press, and the other agencies for the cure and prevention of hookworm disease."[17]

To this initial statement of purpose, Rose added an important caveat in his first annual report. It was not simply desirable, he asserted, but imperative that the Commission discharge its re-sponsibilities in cooperation with existing Southern institutions, for the problem fell within their rightful jurisdiction. The Com-mission could be helpful only insofar as it might call Southerners' attention to the specific need and stimulate them to marshal their own forces against the menace of hookworm. This salient after-thought was certainly in keeping with Gates's and Rockefeller's philosophy of philanthropy. Rose may have thought of hook-worm as the "entering wedge" for public health work in general, but there is no evidence to suggest that he or anyone else in the Rockefeller organization hoped it would also prove to be the Trojan Horse by which they would gain access to, and eventually take over, the South's embryonic public health bureaus. Chapin had wondered whether the benefits accrued from a Rockefeller-sponsored campaign against hookworm were worth the dangers inherent in the financial dependency of state organizations on an outside source. Nothing in the Commission's record, however, led him to conclude that the problem was anything other than poten-tial. Rose was careful to circumscribe direct action on the part of the Commission into the affairs of the people it served. Its labors were undoubtedly more fruitful as a result.

Several closely interrelated objectives grew out of the long-range goals set out in Rockefeller's letter. One of the first, in terms of immediate priority, was to demonstrate to the people of the South that hookworm disease constituted a threat to their well-being; that it was widely prevalent throughout the region and was undermining their health; but, at the same time, that it was easily cured. Rose could state without exaggeration at the conclusion of the Commission's work that this particular goal had been met. Public opinion in 1910 had been dubious, often openly hostile to the announcement of the Commission's formation. The "germ of laziness" was thought to be the invention of a slightly addled Yankee mountebank, taken up by the accursed Rockefel-lers for the humiliation and further discredit of the South. "Yet a golden-tongued orator," as one commentary pointed out, "was hard-pressed to explain away the high incidence of worm eggs found in the stools of people in 35 Alabama counties," for exam-ple.[18] Once the Commission had proved conclusively that hook-worm was one of the facts of Southern life, no responsible person could doubt the wisdom of a campaign to bring about its eradica-tion. It is to the credit of erstwhile unbelievers that they swal-lowed their apprehensions (along with their thymol) as quickly as they did once sufficient evidence was in and either passively ac-quiesced in or wholeheartedly endorsed the work of the Commis-sion. Regarding this aspect of their labors, Rose could conclude: "One may still find individuals here and there who do not take the disease seriously; nevertheless, the Commission may regard this part of its work as done."[19]

A second goal of the Commission in 1910 was to make a reliable survey of the South, county by county, to determine the degree of infection in specific locales and for the region as a whole. This survey was conducted along the lines established at the Atlanta conference of state directors in 1911. The decision to use school-children for the surveys proved to be an excellent one. Most field workers shared the sentiments of Dr. Francis Arthur Bell of the South Carolina corps, who, in response to a 1939 Rockefeller Foundation questionnaire, wrote:

I am still practicing medicine and surgery, and am treating adults now, who were children during the hookworm campaign of 1910. These patients often refer to the days when, with a projection machine, alcohol-lighted, I lectured in the different county churches and schoolhouses on the life cycle and dangers attendant to the Necator Americanus. These adult patients are the children I addressed publically twenty-eight years ago, and they still remember the pertinent points of my lectures and are now putting them to practical use in regards to health measures and sanitation.

In those early days of the fight against hook-worm and soil pollution, it was difficult to get an audience of adults to attend a lecture concerning health matters, but the children attended in full force. These young people would carry the message home to the older ones, who would later question me on matters pertaining to sanitation. In this way, I taught the doubting adults thru the children.

The point I wish to make is that any proved scientific fact that conflicts with local time-worn traditions must be "put over" by intensive education of the children.[20]

By the end of 1914, 548,992 children between the ages of six and eighteen had been examined. The children represented 596 counties, on an average of 921 per county. Of the total number of children examined, 216,828 were found infected, establishing an index of 39 percent by the time the Commission folded. It should be noted that this percentage was down four points from the earlier estimate forecast after two years' work. Since the survey was carried into many new counties in the intervening three years, it is impossible to determine whether the reduction in infection was due to the success of the dispensaries and the cooperation of private physicians or simply the result of introducing the survey into counties with a naturally lighter degree of infection. Whichever explanation is closer to the truth, the absolute index of 39 percent, recorded in 1914, provided a standard against which future surveys could measure progress.[21]

Another of the Commission's original ambitions was to conduct a second survey, this one designed to indicate the condition of soil pollution responsible for the existence of hookworm infection in the first place. Obviously pollution would be greatest in those counties with the highest indexes of infection. The data gathered from this second survey were collated according to Stiles's rather cumbersome rule of thumb, designed to evaluate and rate the South's privies by degree of sanitation. Altogether 250,680 homes were inspected by Stiles and the field workers. Of these 125,584, or roughly 50 percent, were without privies of any sort. Only about 10,000 possessed outhouses that met Stiles's minimum standards. The resulting sanitary index was only 6.3 percent. Here was an area in which much work remained to be done. but the Commission's last report only noted that "the sanitary survey . . . while valuable in [itself], [has] been carried on incidentally to the work of cure and prevention, with very little added expense of time or money."[22] Southern communities began to pass ordinances specifying minimum health standards in the construction and location of privies, but the solution to the soil pollution problem in the rural South awaited the introduction of sewer lines in the small towns and septic tanks on the farms.

The first institution mentioned in the list of agencies in the South through which the Commission hoped to carry out its crusade against the hookworm was the medical profession. The approach here took two forms: first, by helping the practicing physicians recognize and treat the disease, and second, by encouraging instruction in the region's medical schools. Surprisingly, the effort to enlist the South's doctors in support of the Commission's work did not work out as well as Rose had hoped. Despite the personal visits, lectures, letters, and questionnaires, less than a third of the region's physicians reported that they had treated hookworm patients before the end of 1914. In fact, only 13,034 out of 27,407 Southern doctors responded to the Commission's questionnaire at all.[23] Of course there is no way of estimating exactly what percentage of the medical force actually treated the disease; still, only 9,027 responded in the affirmative to the Commission's inquiries. It is hard to imagine a large number of doctors in the South so oblivious to the day-to-day events in their home towns that they knew as little about the hookworm in 1914 as they had in 1910. More substantial progress was made in the area of medical eduction. According to a survey conducted in 1913, 22 of the

South's 29 medical schools were offering as a regular part of their curricula lectures and clinical instruction in hookworm infection. Two schools reported giving incidental instruction, while the other five did not respond. Tulane, the best medical school south of Baltimore at the time, provided a high standard of instruction. In its letter to the Commission, it noted:

Students in the junior year practice the laboratory diagnosis of hookworm disease and other intestinal parasites for ten or twelve hours. These students are thoroughly drilled in the technique, and required to make diagnoses on a large number of specimens.

In the senior year, the students make practical diagnoses of all cases which occur in their service during one-half the term. It is probable that each student performs diagnoses upon from ten to fifty cases of intestinal parasites. In the didactic lectures, two lectures of one hour each are given, in which general symptomatology and the treatment of the disease are thoroughly discussed. In the clinics each student sees from a few up to thirty or forty cases, perhaps, under treatment in his service during the session. It is seldom, however, that a student does not have one or more cases of hookworm disease assigned to him for diagnosis, and to be watched and treated. The fundamental principles of prevention are thoroughly explained, both in the didactic lecture and in the lecture introductory to the laboratory diagnosis.[24]

Although instruction in hookworm disease was more intensive at Tulane than at the other Southern medical schools, the Commission could number as one of its successes the fact that the South would not see another generation of young physicians without some knowledge of hookworm.

The educational campaign to indoctrinate the Southern population in the ways to treat and prevent hookworm infection took up a large portion of the Commission's time and money, and ranked in importance with the therapeutic side of its work from the outset. The educational campaign was waged in almost every corner of Southern life, through practically every medium of communication. The press, the pulpit, the speaker's platform, the mails, and the public schools all joined in the cooperative movement to develop in the Southern people an understanding of the characteristics of the hookworm. The program notes from a 1914 community assembly in Leila, Georgia, give a good idea of one of the many forms such a joint effort could take:

| 1st. | *Piano solo.* | Harriet Martin. |
| 2nd. | *Recitation.* | Fourth Grade. |
| 3rd. | *The house fly and mosquito.* | Dr. E. S. Davis. |

| | | |
|---|---|---|
| 4th. | *Quartette.* | Messrs. Riddick & Davis, Mrs. Herring & Elliott |
| 5th. | *How to have general clean up day.* | Led by Mrs. Stokes and Mrs. Herring. |
| 6th. | *Duet.* | May Gibson & Hattie Lela Davis. |
| 7th. | *Reproduction of Legend of Sleepy Hollow.* | Mr. Fullerton, Jr. |
| 8th. | *Solo.* | Mrs. Bullard. |
| 9th. | *County Home Sanitation.* | Mrs. W. W. Gibson. |
| 10th. | *Song.* | Fourth Grade. |
| 11th. | *Duty of business men toward preserving the health of the community.* | Mr. Cummings & Mrs. Stokes. |
| 12th. | *Quartette.* | Cecil Davis, Sampson Waddell, Raymond Fullerton, and Clarence Waddell. |
| 13th. | *Recitation.* | Ruby Waddell. |
| 14th. | *Disinfecting as a preventative of disease and a promotion of health.* | Led by Mr. Frank Rentz & Dr. Davis. |
| | *Jokes* | W. J. Elliot. |
| 15th. | *Stereopticon lecture on hookworm by special request.* | Dr. A. W. Wood.[25] |

In each county where infection was severe enough to warrant it, the Commission proposed to undertake a systematic drive to saturate the population with lectures, demonstrations, exhibits, and the printed word. The dispensary was an invaluable part of such a campaign. Of the 968 counties in the eleven states,[26] dispensary work was conducted in 578. Almost always, the county itself appropriated several hundred dollars to help finance a dispensary. As a Sparta, Georgia, county commissioner told the field worker for his district: "Well, we have just spent some money to stamp out hog cholera; it seems hookworm might as well go.'[27] (To which Rose replied: "When the people are ready to vote money for the protection of the life of their children as readily as for the protection of their hogs the public health movement is making great progress.")[28] By the end of 1914, 100 counties were still in need of dispensary work. After the dissolution of the Sanitary Commission, the International Health Commission carried on the work in some of these neglected areas.[29]

Work in the public schools centered on instruction in the dangers of soil pollution and the ways to prevent it. Rose concluded that this phase of the educational campaign met with gratifying success but remained far from complete fulfillment in 1914. The school departments served as the Commission's strongest allies in the work. In many cases, the county boards of education appropriated funds to promote local anti-hookworm work. Virginia and Louisiana enacted ordinances requiring the construction and utilization of sanitary privies at all the public schools, and North Carolina refused to approve the plans for a new schoolhouse unless it was to be provided with a safe outhouse. Local boards in many of the other states took similar action on their own accords, although no general measures were adopted by their respective state agencies. Fairly comprehensive instruction on the subject of soil pollution became a regular part of the public school curriculum in Virginia, North Carolina, South Carolina, Georgia, Alabama, Louisiana, Texas, and Kentucky. In Virginia, North Carolina, Alabama, and Kentucky the textbooks used for his purpose were supplemented by bulletins, leaflets, and catechisms prepared by either the Commission or the state boards of health. A bulletin of the U.S. Bureau of Education, issued in 1914, reported that several of the other Southern states, such as Tennessee, Mississippi, and Arkansas, held special health days, under the direction of the local boards of education, for instruction in the ways to improve sanitation.[30]

As important as all these objectives were, they remained peripheral to the main, avowed purpose of the Sanitary Commission to get the sufferers cured. Rose did not hazard a guess at the number of hookworm victims cured by the Commission through its field workers or by private physicians in the course of their practices during the five years of the Commission's life. Nor could he: private physicians were poor correspondents, and patients treated in the dispensaries were not followed up. In this important area, all Rose could cite were the statistics on the number of treatments dispensed, an impressive number in its own right. By the end of 1914, 694,494 Southerners had received at least one dose of thymol and salts—all but 254,118 of them in dispensaries.[31]

The Commission did not find it necessary, probably as the result of both the unexpected financial support of the counties and Rose's stinginess, to spend all of Rockefeller's original gift. Over the course of the five years, it spent a total of $680,023.05 through the various state and county health agencies and another $117,865.31 to defray administrative expenses. The remaining $202,111.64 of the Sanitary Commission's money, along with all its possessions, were turned over to the International Health Commission in January 1915.[32]

What significance can be attached to this welter of goals, achievements, statistics, results, and percentages? Was the Sanitary Commission a success? Did it accomplish what it set out to do? What was its legacy? If one's sole criterion for evaluating its work hinges on the question of eradication, the Commission would have to be considered a failure. Before rushing to judgment, however, the critic of the Commission should pause long enough to consider the fact that the word "eradication" was inserted in the official title of the organization at Gates's insistance, and over Stiles's considered objections, to achieve a psychological effect, even at the expense of realistic expectations based on carefully gathered evidence. Nowhere else – not in Rockefeller's initial letter, not in the Commission's bylaws, not in Rose's list of objectives in the first annual report – does eradication appear as one of the Commission's formal goals. It now seems unlikely that the people of the South would have refused to cooperate with the Commission's agents exclusively on the basis of its title. Gates, inclusion of the word can only be seen, therefore, as a strategic blunder. To anyone familiar with the realities of hookworm infection in the South – and this certainly included the state directors and their staffs – eradication was inconceivable within the five-year time limit and had been from the very beginning. Gates, then, sowed the wind in 1909 by encouraging everyone connected with the work to believe that the Sanitary Commission would be around until hookworm disease was no longer a Southern problem. He reaped the whirlwind five years later when he shut down the Commission before the promise implicit in its title had come close to fulfillment. The Rockefeller Sanitary Commission for the Eradication of Hookworm Disease was not a failure, but its name was ill chosen.

Perhaps the Commission's most important legacy in the South was the network of state and local public health agencies it left in its wake. In 1910, Rose had found the state public health systems understaffed, legally powerless, and without adequate funds. Public opinion regarding the social role of these agencies was also undeveloped. During the Commission's five-year sojourn in the South, all this changed. People developed an unanticipated interest and relative sophistication in matters pertaining to hookworm infection and public health in general. On the state level, this new attitude was reflected in the 81 percent increase in state appropriations for health work between 1910 and 1914. Several state agencies were given the power to promulgate and enforce state-wide health ordinances. In retrospect, most state public health officials agreed with Dr. Watson S. Rankin, Secretary of the North Carolina State Board of Health, who told Rose in 1911 that "the indirect stimulating influence of your commission on state boards of health . . . is in reality the biggest work that you are doing."[33] Fifty-two years later, Rankin had not changed his mind. "I have used Esso gasoline all my life," he told an interviewer, "out of admiration for the Rockefeller Sanitary Commission and what it did. The Rockefeller Foundation had a lot to do with starting full-time public health services in the South."[34] From another angle of vision, the historian C. Vann Woodward observed: "While the public-health awakening in the South clearly antedated the hookworm campaign, it is evident that a tremendous stimulus derived from the . . . work of the Rockefeller Sanitary Commission."[35] In his last report as administrative secretary of the Commission, Rose noted that "it is a matter for congratulation that the co-operative efforts of the Commission and of the State departments of health, exerted in one field – that of hookworm disease – have proved stimulative to other departments of health work, and have aided in the development of public health agencies by the States and communities."[36]

County health bureaus, in the few places where they existed at all before the arrival of the Commission, usually consisted of a part-time doctor who took on the county-wide responsibilities as an adjunct to his regular practice. In February 1911, the North Carolina legislature approved a bill authorizing counties to support full-time health officers and specifically listed as one of his duties the examination of feces for hookworm infection. On June 1, 1911, Guilford county, North Carolina, became the first county in the United States to appoint a full-time health officer and paid him an annual salary of $2,500, twice the starting salary of the Commission's field workers. Guilford county contained a large city – Charlotte – but in 1912, another North Carolina county, Robeson, without a single incorporated place of more than 2,500 people, became the first completely rural county in the country to hire a full-time health officer. In 1910, the combined total of funds appropriated by county organizations for use in public health work amounted to only $241.50. By 1915 the picture was considerably brighter. Rose could conclude that, by the time of the Commission's dissolution, the local agencies had supplied a total of $110,139.79, or $19,773.33 more than the amount spent by the counties for work there. In other words, the participating Southern counties had wiped out an adverse ratio of appropriations to expenditures and established a distinctly favorable one, all within the half-decade of the Commission's life. The financial statistics indicate that, despite the fact that the Commission refused to supplement budgets for general public health work, it did help to create an atmosphere in which such work could begin. In the words of a writer in *The South Atlantic Quarterly*, "the importance of the Rockefeller Commission's work lies in the fact that it is an organized and aggressive campaign for better sanitation in the South."[37] Rose's final word on the subject was optimistic: "It would appear that the hopes of the founder have been largely realized . . . With the awakening public sense, and the growing belief in the fundamental need for preventive measures, the future for public health work seems bright."[38] When the International Health Commission went back into the South several years later, it chose to build on the county public health base that had first been laid down at the time of the Rockefeller Sanitary Commission.[39]

The second important legacy of the Sanitary Commission was its contribution to the early methods and programs of the Rockefeller Foundation. Scholars may reasonably debate whether, on balance, the impact of the Rockefeller Foundation on American life in the twentieth century has been salutary or harmful. The effect itself, however, can hardly be a source of controversy, for it is clearly there for all to see, and it has been profound. So large a hand has the Foundation had in shaping the features of our society that any wholesale indictment of its operational philosophy or practical consequences usually reflects the individual critic's disenchantment with that society itself. Since the Foundation was initially created, and has continued to be nourished, with the first profits from that quintessential twentieth-century industry—petroleum—and since its priorities—research, scientific medicine, public health, and social engineering—mirror the values that might well be used to differentiate our century from the last, it would be easy to lose sight of the fact that its own origins can be traced to an America that it helped to replace. It was conceived shortly after the turn of the century by Gates and the two Rockefellers, who thought they were drawing up a scientific blueprint to promote the well-being of mankind throughout the world. One of the important things that a study of the Sanitary Commission demonstrates, however, is that their instincts were overwhelmingly religious—specifically evangelical. The evidence for this conclusion does not rest on a fuzzy and schematic linkage of vaguely compatible ideas but comes directly and demonstrably from the oftentimes unconscious attitudes and assumptions expressed in the memoirs and correspondence of the Foundation's architects and from an exploration of the model for the Foundation's first efforts—the Sanitary Commission. Although they were not aware of it, Gates and the Rockefellers employed the methods of evangelical Christianity to wage war on hookworm disease, which, in Gates's mind at least, had taken on all the features of the old evangelical notion of sin. If the Sanitary Commission was the tiny acorn from which grew the Rockefeller Foundation itself, then the roots of the Foundation—that most modern of American institutions—lie buried deep in the good, rich, evangelical soil of rural, nineteenth-century America.

# Abbreviations

| | |
|---|---|
| *DSB* | *Dictionary of Scientific Biography*, ed.-in-chief Charles Coulston Gillispie, 15 vols. (New York: Charles Scribner's Sons, 1970-1978). |
| GEB | The General Education Board |
| Hackett MSS | A manuscript history of the International Health Division of the Rockefeller Foundation written by Lewis W. Hackett and housed at the Rockefeller Archive Center, Hillcrest, Pocantico Hills, North Tarrytown, New York. |
| IHC | |
| IHB | |
| IHD | The International Health Commission (also the International Health Board and the International Health Division) of the Rockefeller Foundation. |
| RF | The Rockefeller Foundation |
| RI | The Rockefeller Institute for Medical Research (now the Rockefeller University) |
| RSC | The Rockefeller Sanitary Commission for the Eradication of Hookworm Disease |
| RSC Coll. | The Rockefeller Sanitary Commission Collection, Rockefeller Archive Center |
| SEB | The Southern Education Board |

# Notes

## Prologue

1. Robert Penn Warren, *The Legacy of the Civil War* (New York: Knopf, 1961), p. 57.

2. Thomas D. Clark, *The Emerging South* (New York: Oxford University Press, 1961), p. 24.

3. W. J. Cash, *The Mind of the South* (New York: Knopf, 1941), p. 37.

4. Clark, *The Emerging South*, p. 26.

5. Harold W. Brown, *Basic Clinical Parasitology*, 4th ed. (New York: Appleton-Century-Crofts, 1975), pp. 121-129; Paul E. Beeson and Walsh McDermott, *Texbook of Medicine*, 14th ed. (Philadelphia: W. B. Saunders Co., 1975), pp. 524-526.

6. Marcel Roche and Miguel Layrisse, "The Nature and Causes of 'Hookworm Anemia,'" *American Journal of Tropical Medicine and Hygiene*, 15 (November 1966), 1052-1053. See also H. M. Gilles, E. J. Watson Williams, and P. A. J. Ball, "Hookworm Infection and Anaemia," *Quarterly Journal of Medicine*, n.s. 33 (January 1964), 18; and Norman R. Stoll, "For Hookworm Diagnosis, Is Finding an Egg Enough?" *Annals of the New York Academy of Sciences*, 98 (August 31, 1962), 712-724 ("adequately nourished hosts are themselves able to deal with minor infestations," p. 713).

7. Roche and Layrisse, "Hookworm Anemia," p. 1053.

8. Brown, *Clinical Parasitology*, p. 126. See also Todd L. Savitt, *Medicine and Slavery: The Diseases and Health Care of Blacks in Antebellum Virginia* (Urbana: University of Illinois Press, 1978), pp. 46, 69-71. The "discoverer of hookworm disease" in the United States, Charles Wardell Stiles, addressed himself to the question of black susceptibility in his *Hookworm Disease and Its Relation to the Negro* (Washington: Government Printing Office, 1909).

9. Benjamin E. Washburn, *As I Recall* (New York: RF, 1960), p. 4.

10. RSC, publication no. 5, *Second Annual Report* (Washington: RSC, 1911), p. 120.

11. Joan Bicknell, *Pica: A Childhood Symptom* (London: Butter-

worths, 1975), pp. 4, 91-94; Robert W. Twyman, "The Clay Eater: A New look at an Old Southern Enigma," *Journal of Southern History*, 27 (August 1971), 443-447.

12. Thymol is a phenol (carbolic acid) that may either be extracted from the herb thyme ("thyme-oil") or synthesized in a laboratory. Presented to the patient as either "colorless crystals or white, crystalline powder," thymol was first used as a disinfectant and later as a fungicide. When taken as a vermifuge, "it had to be used in such large doses that there was danger of serious, even fatal, poisioning." When swallowed, some of its disquieting side effects include "nausea, vomiting . . . headache, ringing in the ears, dizziness, muscular weakness, thready pulse, slow respiration, and fall of body temperature. The heart is depressed by 'therapeutic' doses." See Arthur Osol and Robertson Pratt, *The United States Dispensatory*, 27th ed. (Philadelphia: J. B. Lippincott, 1973), pp. 1189-1190.

## 1. Charles Wardell Stiles

1. Randolph Bourne, "American Use for German Ideals," *New Republic*, September 4, 1915, p. 118.

2. Ibid., p. 117.

3. Several sources provide biographical information on Stiles: Charles Wardell Stiles, "Early History, in Part Esoteric, of the Hookworm (Uncinariasis) Campaign in Our Southern States," *Journal of Parasitology*, 25 (August 1939), 283-308, an autobiographical account which picks up his career in 1891; Mark Sullivan, *Our Times, 1900–1925*, 6 vols. (New York: Charles Scribner's Sons, 1930), III, 299-303, proofread and amended by Stiles before publication; Frank G. Brooks, "Charles Wardell Stiles, Intrepid Scientist," *Bios*, 18 (1947), 139-169, written using information furnished in part by Stiles to the author; Charles Wardell Stiles, *National Cyclopedia of American Biography*, current vol. D (New York: James T. White and Co., 1934), pp. 62-63; Benjamin Schwartz, "A Brief Resumé of Dr. Stiles' Contributions to Parasitology," *Journal of Parasitology*, 19 (June 1933), 257-261; James H. Cassedy, "Charles Wardell Stiles," in *DSB*, XIII, 62-63.

4. Brooks, "Stiles," p. 139.

5. Ibid., pp. 140-143.

6. George M. Beard, the late-nineteenth-century New York physician, was widely regarded as the clinician chiefly responsible for describing the disorder, or state of mental agitation, known as "neurasthenia." As a young man, Beard had suffered a crisis that closely resembled Stiles's. Beard too had wanted to study medicine; his father and grand-father, like Stiles's were ministers. See Barbara Sicherman, "The Uses of a Diagnosis: Doctors, Patients, and Neurasthenia," *Journal of the History of Medicine and Allied Sciences*, 32 (January 1977), 33-54; see also Charles E. Rosenberg, *No Other Gods: On Science and American Social Thought* (Baltimore: The John Hopkins University Press, 1976), chap. 5.

7. Brooks, "Stiles," p. 144.

8. Ibid., pp. 144-147; Thomas Neville Bonner, *American Doctors and German Universities* (Lincoln: University of Nebraska Press, 1963), p. 84; Daniel J. Kevles, *The Physicists: The History of a Scientific Community in Modern America* (New York: Knopf, 1977), pp. 15-16; R. Steven Turner, "Hermann von Helmholtz," *DSB*, VI, 241-253; Paul Glees, "Wilhelm von Waldeyer-Hartz," *DSB*, XIV, 125-126.

9. Brooks, "Stiles," p. 147; K. E. Rothschuh, "Emil Heinrich du Bois-Reymond," *DSB*, XIV, 200-205.

10. Brooks, "Stiles," p. 147.

11. Quoted in H. Schadewaldt, "Karl Georg Friedrich Rudolf Leuckart," *DSB*, XIII, 270.

12. Ibid., pp. 269-271; E. M. Pantelouris, *The Common Liver Fluke* (New York: Pergamon Press, 1965), pp. 9-10.

13. Brooks, "Stiles," p. 147.

14. Ibid., pp. 147-148; James H. Cassedy, "Applied Microscopy and American Pork Diplomacy: Charles Wardell Stiles in Germany, 1898–1899," *Isis*, 62 (Spring 1971), 8, n. 10; Charles Wardell Stiles, "Notes sur les parasites. I. Sur la dent des embryons d'Ascaris," *Bulletin de la Société Zoologique de France*, 16 (1891), 162-163.

15. Brooks, "Stiles," pp. 149-151; Gert H. Brieger, "Elie Metchnikoff," *DSB*, IX, 331-335.

16. Brooks, "Stiles," p. 151; Schwartz, "A Brief Resumé," p. 261; Cassedy, "Applied Microscopy," p. 8.

17. Schwartz, "A Brief Resumé," pp. 257-258; Cassedy, "Applied Microscopy," p. 8.

18. Brooks, "Stiles," pp. 167-169; Cassedy, "Applied Microscopy," p. 10.

19. Quoted in James H. Cassedy, "The 'Germ of Laziness' in the South, 1901–1915: Charles Wardell Stiles and the Progressive Paradox," *Bulletin of the History of Medicine*, 45 (March-April 1971), 161.

## 2. The Scientist as Lone Evangelist

1. Pierce's statement is from the message accompanying his veto of a bill, inspired by the work of Dorothea Dix, that would have set aside revenues from the sale of public lands to be used for the care of the insane. It is quoted in Robert H. Bremner, *American Philanthropy* (Chicago: University of Chicago Press, 1960), p. 70.

2. Stiles, in 1939, compiled a list of over 130 names used to describe hookworm disease. Only 32 are obviously derived from a taxonomic familiarity with the parasite itself. The rest, such as *Geophagia* and *Langue blanche*, describe, often in graphic colloquial terms, the physical symptoms.

3. R. Hoeppli, *Parasites and Parasitic Infections in Early Medicine and Science* (Singapore: Malaya University Press, 1959), p. 493; RF, IHB, publication no. 11, *Bibliography of Hookworm Disease* (New York: RF, 1922), p. xi.

4. RF, IHB, publication no. 11, *Bibliography*, p. xii; Sullivan, *Our Times*, III, 302-303.

5. The Greek letter "gamma" is commonly transliterated as the letter *n* followed by a "chi" sound (usually "ch," as in "anchor"). Dubini chose the letters *g* and *y* instead of either the "nch" or the "nk" combinations.

6. Angelo Dubini, "Nuovo verme intestinale umano (Agychylostoma duodenale) constituente un sesto genere dei nematoidei proprii dell'uomo," *Annali Universale di Medicina e Chirugia*, 106 (1843), 5-13.

7. RF, IHB, publication no. 11, *Bibliography*, p. xiii; Battista Grassi, Corrado Parona, and Ernesto Parona, "Interno a'll Anchilostoma Duodenale (Dubini)," *Gazetta Medica Lombarda*, 7th ser. 5 (1878), 193-196.

8. RF, IHB, publication no. 11, *Bibliography*, pp. xiii-xiv.

9. August Hirsch, *Handbook of Geographical and Historical Pathology*, 3 vols. (London: New Sydenham Society, 1883-1886), translated from the second German edition by Charles Creighton; see II, 313-323.

10. Stiles, "Early History," pp. 285-286.

11. Quoted at greater length in Stiles, "Early History," p. 287.

12. Cassedy, "Applied Microscopy," p. 8.

13. Sullivan, *Our Times*, III, 303-304; W. L. Blickhahn, "Case of Ankylostomiasis," *Medical News*, 63 (December 9, 1893), 662-663; Frank Herff, "Report of Parasite Entozoa Encountered in General Practice in Texas During Over Forty Years," *Texas Medical Journal*, 9 (June 1894), 613-616; F. G. Möhlau, "Anchylostamum [*sic*] duodenale, with report of cases," *Buffalo Medical Journal*, 36 (March 1897), 573-579.

14. Mary Boccaccio, "Ground Itch and Dew Poison: The Rockefeller Sanitary Commission, 1909-14," *Journal of the History of Medicine and Allied Sciences*, 27 (January 1972), 30-31; Stiles, "Early History," p. 289.

15. Probably the most thorough account of German-American relations in the 1890s is to be found in Alfred Vagts, *Deutschland und die Vereinigten Staaten in der Weltpolitik*, 2 vols. (London: L. Dickson and Thompson, 1935); for a good account of the pork boycott, with Stiles as the center of attention, see Cassedy, "Applied Microscopy," pp. 5-20.

16. Stiles married Virginia Baker in June 1897. See Brooks, "Stiles," p. 169.

17. Stiles, "Early History," p. 289; Wilhelm Zinn and Martin Jacoby, *Anchylostomum duodenale: Über seine geographische Verbreitung und seine Bedeutung für die Pathologie* (Leipzig, 1898), pp. 24-51.

18. Bailey K. Ashford, *A Soldier in Science* (New York: W. Morrow & Co., 1934), pp. 1-7, 42-43.

19. Bailey K. Ashford, "Ankylostomiasis in Puerto Rico," *New York Medical Journal*, 71 (April 14, 1900), 552-556.

20. Ashford, *A Soldier in Science*, pp. 46-47.

21. The first official consignment of hookworms from Puerto Rico, lot no. 3437, was collected by Ashford on June 11, 1902, and examined by Stiles on November 25, 1902. This information was provided to Stiles some time in the mid-1930s (after the appearance of Ashford's autobiography and before the publication of Stiles, "Early History") by Dr. Mau-

rice C. Hall from the Catalogue of the Zoological Division, Bureau of Animal Industry. See Stiles, "Early History," p. 293. See also Stiles to W. G. Smillie, June 6, 1938, cited in Hackett MSS, chap. 3, p. 6.

22. Hackett MSS, chap. 3, p. 7; Allen J. Smith, "Uncinariasis in Texas,"*American Journal of Medical Sciences*, n.s. 126 (1903), 768-798; Stiles, "Early History," pp. 292-293; Greer Williams, *The Plague Killers* (New York: Charles Scribner's Sons, 1969), p. 12.

23. Stiles, "Early History," p. 292.

24. A similar anthropological sideshow proved a boon to another hookworm doctor in this period. While stationed in New York in 1902, Bailey Ashford found the disease rife among a group of "authentic Puerto Ricans" imported by an enterprising promoter to inhabit a "typical Puerto Rican village" constructed on Long Island. In the opinion of the somewhat bemused Ashford, the village was far more typical than the entrepreneur had envisioned. See Ashford, *A Soldier in Science*, p. 49.

25. Hackett MSS, chap. 3, p. 8; Arthur Looss, "Note on Intestinal Worms Found in African Pygmies," *The Lancet*, II for 1905 (August 12, 1905), 430-431.

26. Cassedy, "Germ of Laziness," p. 163; Stiles, "Early History," pp. 295-296.

27. C. W. Stiles, "Report upon the Prevalence and Geographic Distribution of Hookworm Disease (Uncinariasis or Anchylostomiasis) in the United States," *United States Public Health Service, Hygienic Laboratory*, Bulletin no. 10 (February 1903), partially reprinted in Sullivan, *Our Times*, III, 314.

28. C. W. Stiles, "Preliminary Report," October 26, 1902, partially reprinted in Williams, *The Plague Killers*, p. 15.

29. H. F. Harris, "Ankylostomiasis, the Most Common of the Serious Diseases in the Southern Part of the United States," *American Medicine*, 4 (1902), 776, quoted in Stiles, "Early History," pp. 294-295.

30. *New York Sun*, December 5, 1902; Sullivan, *Our Times*, III, 290-294; Stiles, "Early History," p. 296; Hacket MSS, chap. 3, pp. 8-9.

31. At the turn of the century, according to the science editor of the Scripps-Howard newspaper chain, "the newspapers had no interest in the reporting of science. Those were the days when a scientific convention was regarded as an assignment for the staff humorist. There were two accepted and traditional methods of reporting such a convention. One was to comment upon the length and luxuriousness of the beards worn by the assembled savants, the other was to make a collection of those titles of papers which contained the longest words and the ones least familiar to the ordinary reader."

The scientists, on their part, viewed the newspapers only with hostility and disdain. They asked nothing better than to be left alone to carry on their deliberations in quietness and privacy." David Dietz, "Science and the American Press," *Science*, 85 (January 29, 1937), 107-108.

32. The first poem was originally published in *Truth*; the editorial, in

the *Salt Lake City Herald*, December 9, 1902; both were reprinted in Sullivan, *Our Times*, III, 297-299.

33. Quoted in Sullivan, *Our Times*, III, 299.

34. Stiles, "Early History," p. 296.

35. In 1898 Looss noticed that his hands began to itch shortly after he had accidentally spilled a hookworm culture on them. When he discovered hookworm ova in his feces, he suspected a dermal infection. His later experiments established both an accurate life cycle for the hookworm as well as the intricate migratory route that the parasite followed through the human body. His theories soon proved superior to several competing explanations and answered the last remaining purely parasitological question about *Uncinaria*. It had been Looss, then, who had discovered not only the internal, physiological path of the parasite but also its historical-geographical vector from Africa to the Western Hemisphere. See Arthur Looss, *The Anatomy and Life History of Agychylostoma Duodenale Dubini*, 2 parts (Cairo: National Printing Department, 1905-1911), translated from the German manuscript by Matilda Bernard.

36. Stiles, "Early History," p. 298.

37. Ibid., p. 297.

38. Ibid., pp. 297-298. There are several interesting points of comparison between the careers of Wiley and Stiles. Wiley had also been brought up in an evangelical home. After studying medicine and chemistry in the United States, he toured the German universities and worked for a time in the German Imperial Health Office. Shortly after accepting a position in 1883 as the chief chemist of the Department of Agriculture, he began his campaign for legislation to control food adulteration and patent medicines. According to James Harvey Young, Wiley "applied his moral fervor to the pure food crusade . . . Like an itinerant preacher, he stumped up and down the country." Even so, Wiley's message failed to move the general public to seek legislative redress until it was restated in 1905 by the journalist Samuel Hopkins Adams in the pages of the muckraking magazine, *Collier's*. Within nine months of the first *Collier's* article, Theodore Roosevelt signed the Pure Food and Drugs Act.

It would be tempting to attribute Wiley's success and Stiles's frustrations to their very different personalities. "Wiley," according to Young, "had a light touch and a warm heart. His wit was the talk of the banquet circuit, and he had a gift for clever doggerel." Although Wiley was certainly no Almus Pickerbaugh, one is reminded of the municipal health officer in *Arrowsmith* whose genial *pousse-café* manner and public health jingles made him so popular that he was eventually elected to Congress. About Wiley, Young continues: "A bachelor, he was free to move about, and he was an ardent clubman, an eager dinner guest. Wiley had the knack of eliciting tremendous loyalty, and his personal associations, tending toward the conspiratorial, were to be as important as his public speaking in the ultimate success of a pure food bill."

Stiles was never as adept at winning friends and charming audiences.

But it should be remembered that Wiley, despite his social gifts, had to work hard for over twenty years before he saw his bill enacted into law. The fact that there was never a federally sponsored campaign against hookworm disease probably has less to do with Stiles's inability to cajole Congressmen than with the perceived difference in the natures of the two threats. Young again: "Wiley's message was not primarily one of fear, for he did not believe that adulteration posed a grave danger to the public health. But his sense of righteousness was offended by fraud, and he inveighed against adulterators as economic cheats." Progressive hackles were more easily raised, it seems, by human parasites than by parasites in humans. See James Harvey Young, *The Toadstool Millionaires: A Social History of Patent Medicines in America before Federal Regulation* (Princeton: Princeton University Press, 1961), pp. 231-232. See also Oscar E. Anderson, Jr., *The Health of a Nation: Harvey W. Wiley and the Fight for Pure Food* (Chicago: University of Chicago Press, 1958).

39. Stiles, "Early History," pp. 288-289. Osler later invited Stiles to contribute to subsequent editions of his textbook. See Sir William Osler and Thomas McGae, eds., *Modern Medicine: Its Theory and Practice*, 2nd ed., rev., (Philadelphia & New York: Lea & Febiger, 1914), which includes C. W. Stiles, "Diseases Caused by Animal Parasites (Exclusive of Protozoan Infections)."

40. Hackett MSS, chap. 3, p. 10.

41. Ibid., chap. 3, pp. 10-11; Stiles, "Early History," p. 297.

42. Greer Williams interview with Benjamin E. Washburn, September 30, 1963, in Greer Williams Notes, RF Archives; Robert H. Wiebe, *The Search for Order, 1877–1920* (New York: Hill and Wang, 1967), chap. 5; James G. Burrow, *Organized Medicine in the Progressive Era: The Move toward Monopoly* (Baltimore: The Johns Hopkins University Press, 1977).

43. Stiles, "Early History," p. 297.

44. See the file of correspondence from Stiles to Wickliffe Rose, RSC Coll.

45. Stiles, "Early History," pp. 297, 299; *New York Sun*, December 5, 1902.

46. This quotation expresses Stiles's opinion of the scientific publications that appeared after a tick scare in the early 1900s. It is taken from Charles W. Stiles, "Zoological Pitfalls for the Pathologist," The Middleton Goldsmith Lecture delivered to the New York Pathological Society, November 30, 1904, pp. 15-17. It is cited in Cassedy, "Germ of Laziness," p. 162.

47. Woodward: "Part of the millowner's resentment toward the humanitarians was his indignation against the presumptions of a rival, for he continued to regard himself as the only philanthropist worthy of the name. It was the philanthropy of the fief, a village privately owned and policed." C. Vann Woodward, *Origins of the New South*, 1877–1913 (Baton Rouge: Louisiana State University Press, 1951), p. 420.

48. Ibid., p. 420; United States Senate, 61st Congress, 2nd Session,

*Report on Condition of Women and Child Wage Earners in the United States*, Document 645, xvii; C. W. Stiles, "Hookworm Disease among Cotton Mill Operatives" in the same *Report* (Washington: Government Printing Office, 1912), p. 10; Boccaccio, "Ground Itch and Dew Poison," p. 34.

49. Woodward, *Origins of the New South*, p. 238; Stiles, "Early History," p. 298.

50. Woodward has marshaled the statistics from the federal census to point up the magnitude of the problem in the South Atlantic states: "In 1900 three out of ten workers in the mills of the South were children under sixteen years of age, and 57.6 per cent of those children were between ten and thirteen. Those under ten, of whom there were many, were not enumerated. A former president of the American Cotton Manufacturers' Association declared that the adoption of an age limit of fourteen would close every mill in North Carolina, because 75 per cent of the spinners in that state were fourteen or younger; the preceding president of the Association estimated that only 30 per cent of the cotton-mill operatives of the South were adults over twenty-one years of age." Woodward, *Origins of the New South*, p. 416. At the turn of the century no Southern state had a child-labor law among its statues; in 1895 Alabama had rescinded its very mild one at the insistence of a Massachusetts company that was considering locating a mill there.

51. Ibid., p. 419.

52. Ibid.

53. Boccaccio, "Ground Itch and Dew Poison," pp. 33-35; Stiles, "Early History," p. 299.

## 3. Frederick T. Gates and the Business of Benevolence

1. Charles W. Stiles to J. A. Ferrell, February 3, 1939, RSC Coll.

2. All of the Andrew Carnegie quotations are from his article "Wealth," *North American Review*, 148 (June 1889), 653-664.

3. George M. Frederickson, *The Inner Civil War: Northern Intellectuals and the Crisis of the Union* (New York: Harper & Row, 1965), chaps. 6, 7, 12, 13; Bremner, *American Philanthropy*, pp. 80-104.

4. The letter from Rockefeller to Carnegie is quoted in Burton J. Hendrick, *The Life of Andrew Carnegie*, 2 vols. (Garden City, N.Y.: Doubleday, Doran, and Co., 1932), I, 349.

5. Allan Nevins, *John D. Rockefeller: The Heroic Age of American Enterprise*, 2 vols. (New York: Charles Scribner's Sons, 1940), I, 105-107.

6. Mencken's observation is quoted in Peter Collier and David Horowitz, *The Rockefellers: An American Dynasty* (New York: Holt, Rinehart and Winston, 1976), p. 37.

7. Bernard Bailyn, ed., *The Apologia of Robert Keayne* (New York: Harper & Row, 1964), pp. 75-76.

8. John D. Rockefeller, *Random Reminiscences of Men and Events* (New York: Doubleday, Page, and Co., 1909), p. 143.

9. Nevins, *John D. Rockefeller*, I, chaps. 1-6; John K. Winkler, *John D. Rockefeller: A Portrait in Oils* (New York: Vanguard Press, 1929), p. 12; Collier and Horowitz, *The Rockefellers*, p. 8.

10. Collier and Horowitz, *The Rockefellers*, pp. 9-10; Rockefeller, *Random Reminiscences,* pp. 134-136.

11. The Cotton Mather quotation is cited in Bremner, *American Philanthropy*, p. 14.

12. Collier and Horowitz, *The Rockefellers*, p. 10; Rockefeller, *Random Reminiscences*, pp. 146, 154. "The progressive era is almost made to order for the study of Americans in love with efficiency. For the progressive era gave rise to an efficiency craze – a secular Great Awakening, an outpouring of ideas and emotions in which a gospel of efficiency was preached without embarrassment to businessmen, workers, doctors, housewives, and teachers, and yes, preached even to preachers. Men as disparate as William Jennings Bryan and Walter Lippmann discoursed enthusiastically on efficiency. Efficient and good came closer to meaning the same thing in these years than in any other period of American history." See Samuel Haber, *Efficiency and Uplift: Scientific Management in the Progressive Era*, 1890–1920 (Chicago: University of Chicago Press, 1964), p. ix.

13. Ida Tarbell, *The History of the Standard Oil Company*, 2 vols. (New York: McClure, Phillips & Co., 1904), II, 141.

14. Allan Nevins, *Study in Power: John D. Rockefeller, Industrialist and Philanthropist*, 2 vols. (New York: Charles Scribner's Sons, 1953), II, 301.

15. This quotation is reprinted in Nevins, *John D. Rockefeller*, II, 266-267.

16. Collier and Horowitz, *The Rockefellers*, p. 59.

17. Frederick Taylor Gates, *Chapters in My Life* (New York: The Free Press, 1977), p. 161. Written towards the end of his life for private distribution among members of his family, Gates's autobiography remained in manuscript form in the RF Archives until 1977.

18. Ibid., p. 161.

19. Ibid., pp. 17-18.

20. Ibid., p. 35.

21. Ibid., pp. 45-46, 53-54.

22. Ibid., pp. 50-56.

23. Anderson may well have fallen victim to "ministers' sore throat," a rather mysterious but commonplace occupational affliction in the decades before the Civil War. See James H. Cassedy, "An American Clerical Crisis: Ministers' Sore Throat, 1830–1860," *Bulletin of the History of Medicine*, 53 (Spring 1979), 23-38.

24. *The National Cyclopedia of American Biography*, XII (New York, 1904), pp. 243-244.

25. Gates, *Chapters in My Life*, p. 71.

26. Ibid., pp. 65-66.

27. Ibid., p. 72.

28. Ibid., p. 130.

29. Ibid., p. 123.

30. Ibid., pp. 77-81.

31. Ibid., p. 76.

32. Ibid., pp. 83-88.

33. Ibid., p. 114.

34. Ibid., pp. 97-121; Nevins, *Study in Power*, II, chaps. 28, 29.

35. Gates, *Chapters in My Life*, p. 123.

36. Ibid., p. 131.

37. Ibid., pp. 161-162; Frederickson, *The Inner Civil War*, pp. 213-215; Nevins, *Study in Power*, II, chap. 30.

38. Gates, *Chapters in My Life*, p. 165.

39. Nevins, *John D. Rockefeller*, II, 212.

40. Rockefeller, *Random Reminiscences*, p. 117.

41. Gates, *Chapters in My Life*, pp. 165-167, 174.

42. Rockefeller, *Random Reminiscences*, pp. 120-132; Nevins, *John D. Rockefeller*, II, 360-426; Collier and Horowitz, *The Rockefellers*, pp. 54-56; Gates, *Chapters in My Life*, pp. 176-177.

43. Gates, *Chapters in My Life*, p. 206.

44. Quoted in Nevins, *John D. Rockefeller*, II, 281.

45. Ibid.

46. Rockefeller, *Random Reminiscences*, p. 117.

47. B. C. Forbes, "John D. Rockefeller Tells How to Succeed," *Forbes Magazine*, September 29, 1917, p. 69.

48. Gates, *Chapters in My Life*, p. 210.

49. Frederick T. Gates to Dr. Charles W. Eliot, December 30, 1910, RF Archives.

50. Raymond Fosdick, *The Story of the Rockefeller Foundation* (New York: Harper & Brothers, 1952), p. 2.

51. Nevins, *Study in Power*, II, 214.

52. Raymond Fosdick, *John D. Rockefeller, Jr.: A Portrait* (New York: Harper & Brothers, 1956), pp. 111-112.

## 4. Philanthropy for the Ages

1. Gates, *Chapters in My Life*, p. 181.

2. The most comprehensive account of the early negotiations leading to the creation of the Rockefeller Institute for Medical Research may be found in George W. Corner, *A History of the Rockefeller Institute, 1901–1953: Origins and Growth* (New York: RI Press, 1964). Information in this paragraph is in chap. 1.

3. The two biographies of Welch are Simon and James Thomas Flexner, *William Henry Welch and the Heroic Age of American Medicine* (New York: Viking Press, 1941), and Donald Fleming, *William Henry Welch and the Rise of Modern Medicine* (Boston: Little, Brown & Co., 1954).

4. Biographical information on Flexner has been taken from George

W. Corner, "Simon Flexner," *Dictionary of American Biography*, eds. John A. Garraty and Edward T. James, supplement 4 (New York: Charles Scribner's Sons, 1974), 286-289; George W. Corner, "Simon Flexner," *DSB*, V, 39-41; Gates, *Chapters in My Life*, pp. 183-184.

5. Daniel Boorstin, *The Americans: The Democratic Experience* (New York: Random House, 1973), p. 49.

6. Quoted in Corner, *Rockefeller Institute*, p. 154.

7. Gates, *Chapters in My Life*, pp. 205-206.

8. Ibid., pp. 187-188.

9. Ibid., p. 188.

10. Ibid.

11. Ibid., pp. 186-187.

12. Twelfth Census, 1900, *Population*, II, ciii-cv, cited in Woodward, *Origins of the New South*, p 400.

13. See Willie Lee Rose, *Rehearsal for Reconstruction: The Port Royal Experiment* (New York: Knopf, 1964).

14. For information on the Peabody Fund and on George Peabody, see Jabez L. M. Curry, *A Brief Sketch of George Peabody and a History of the Peabody Education Fund through Thirty Years* (New York: Negro Universities Press, 1969), originally published in 1898; Hoy Taylor, *An Interpretation of the Early Administration of the Peabody Education Fund*, in George Peabody College for Teachers, *Contributions to Education*, no. 114 (Nashville: George Peabody College, 1933).

15. Taylor, *An Interpretation of the Early Administration of the Peabody Fund*, pp. 20-21.

16. For information on the Slater Fund, see Ullin W. Leavell, *Philanthropy in Negro Education*, in George Peabody College for Teachers, *Contributions to Education*, no. 100 (Nashville: George Peabody College, 1930); and Henry A. Bullock, *A History of Negro Education in the South from 1619 to the Present* (Cambridge, Mass.: Harvard University Press, 1967).

17. Fosdick, *Rockefeller Foundation*, p. 9; Raymond Fosdick, *Adventure in Giving: The Story of the General Education Board, A Foundation Established by John D. Rockefeller* (New York: Harper & Row, 1962), p. 5. Fosdick's *Adventure in Giving* is based on an unfinished manuscript prepared by Henry F. and Katherine Douglas Pringle.

18. Fosdick and Pringle, *Adventure in Giving*, p. 407; *Proceedings of the Fourth Conference for Education in the South* (n.p., 1901), p. 12; Wickliffe Rose, "The Education Movement in the South," in *Report of the Commissioner of Education for the Year 1903* (Washington: Government Printing Office, 1904), I, 359-390.

19. Charles W. Dabney, "A Brief Statement Concerning the Origin and Organization of the Southern Education Board," in Charles W. Dabney, *Universal Education in the South*, 2 vols. (Chapel Hill: University of North Carolina Press, 1936), II, appendix v, 538-541; *The General Education Board: An Account of Its Activities, 1902–1914* (New York: GEB, 1915), pp. 11-12, 179-180; Fosdick and Pringle, *Adventure in Giving*, pp.

6-7; see also *Southern Education Board: Activities and Results, 1904–1910* (Washington: SEB, 1911).

20. Fosdick and Pringle, *Adventure in Giving*, p. 7.

21. Ray Stannard Baker, *Following the Color Line: An Account of Negro Citizenship in the American Democracy* (New York: Doubleday, Page & Co., 1908), p. 247.

22. Fosdick, *John D. Rockefeller, Jr.*, pp. 116-119; Fosdick and Pringle, *Adventure in Giving*, p. 8; *The General Education Board*, pp. 3-4, appendix ii, 216-218.

23. *The General Education Board*, appendix i, pp. 212-215, 15-17; Fosdick and Pringle, *Adventure in Giving*, appendix i, pp. 327, 22.

24. *The National Cyclopedia of American Biography*, XXII (New York: James T. White & Co., 1932), 419-420; *The General Education Board*, p. 10; Nevins, *Study in Power*, II, 315.

25. Fosdick and Pringle, *Adventure in Giving*, p. 22.

26. Ibid., pp. 21-23.

27. Nevins, *Study in Power*, II, 329.

28. Wallace Buttrick to Edwin A. Alderman, April 1, 1905, in GEB files, Rockefeller Archives Center, quoted in Fosdick and Pringle, *Adventure in Giving*, p. 27.

29. *The General Education Board*, p. 90.

30. Ibid., p. 90.

31. Ibid., pp. 81-86.

32. Fosdick and Pringle, *Adventure in Giving*, p. 40.

33. Ibid., p. 39.

34. Joseph Cannon Bailey, *Seaman A. Knapp: Schoolmaster of American Agriculture* (New York: Columbia University Press, 1945), p. 155.

35. Ibid., p. 157.

36. Seaman A. Knapp, "Improved Conditions for the Southern Farmer," Address at the 10th Conference for Education in the South, Pinehurst, N.C., 1907, quoted in Bailey, *Seaman A. Knapp*, p. 209.

37. Department of Agriculture, *Yearbook, 1903* (Washington: Government Printing Office, 1904), pp 205-208; Bailey, *Seaman A. Knapp*, p. 169; Fosdick and Pringle, *Adventure in Giving*, pp. 41, 43.

38. Fosdick and Pringle, *Adventure in Giving*, pp. 43-45; Bailey, *Seaman A. Knapp*, pp. 217-219; Gates, *Chapters in My Life*, p. 222.

39. Gates, *Chapters in My Life*, pp. 222, 223.

40. Richard Hofstadter, *The Age of Reform: From Bryan to F.D.R.* (New York: Knopf, 1955), p. 119.

## 5. Wickliffe Rose Launches the Sanitary Commission

1. William L. Bowers, *The Country Life Movement in America, 1900–1920* (Port Washington, N.Y.: Kennikat Press, 1974), p. 24.

2. *Washington Post*, November 10, 1908, p. 11.

3. Bowers, *Country Life Movement*, pp. 24-25.

4. Ibid., p. 25; Clayton Ellsworth, "Theodore Roosevelt's Country Life Commission," *Agricultural History*, 34 (October 1960), 161-162.

5. Bowers, *Country Life Movement*, pp. 25-26; Ellsworth, "Roosevelt's Country Life Commission," p. 163.

6. Fleming, *William H. Welch*, pp. 34, 54, 134-135; Hackett MSS, chap. 3, pp. 21-22.

7. Sullivan, *Our Times*, III, 319-320; see also Stiles, "Early History," p. 300; and Burton J. Hendrick, *The Training of an American: The Earlier Life and Letters of Walter H. Page, 1855-1913* (Cambridge, Mass.: Houghton Mifflin, The Riverside Press, 1928), pp. 369-372.

8. Sullivan, *Our Times*, III, 321-323; Burton J. Hendrick, *The Life and Letters of Walter H. Page*, 3 vols. (Garden City, N.Y.: Doubleday, Page & Co., 1923-1925, I, 371.

9. *Washington Post*, November 13, 1908, p. 11.

10. Untitled article draft in Page's handwriting dated October 26, 1909, in the Walter Hines Page Papers, Houghton Library, Harvard University.

11. *Washington Post*, November 21, 1908, p. 1.

12. Hackett MSS, chap. 3, p. 23; Sullivan, *Our Times*, III, 324.

13. Gates, *Chapters in My Life*, p. 225.

14. Hackett MSS, chap. 3, p. 24.

15. Ibid., pp. 23-24; Sullivan, *Our Times*, III, 324; Williams, *The Plague Killers*, pp. 21-22; Stiles, "Early History," p. 301; Gates, *Chapters in My Life*, p. 225.

16. Gates, *Chapters in My Life*, pp. 225-226.

17. Ibid., pp. 226-227.

18. Stiles, "Early History," p. 301.

19. Williams, *The Plague Killers*, p. 23; Stiles, "Early History," p. 301-302.

20. Woodward, *Origins of the New South*, pp. 350, 375.

21. Stiles, "Early History," pp. 301-302.

22. Hackett MSS, chap. 3, p. 29.

23. Frederick T. Gates to Wickliffe Rose, December 17, 1909, RSC Coll.

24. Minutes, meeting of the Board of Directors, RSC, January 15, 1910, p. 13, RSC Coll.

25. John D. Rockefeller to the members of the original board of directors of the RSC, October 26, 1909, RSC Coll.

26. Two members – Joyner and Claxton – were unable to attend the October 26, 1909 meeting.

27. The members of the original board of directors of the RSC to John D. Rockefeller, October 26, 1909, RSC Coll.

28. Article draft dated October 26, 1909, in the Walter Hines Page Papers.

29. Fredrickson, *The Inner Civil War*, p. 102.

30. Ibid., p. 108.

31. Article II, By-Laws of the RSC, RSC Coll.
32. Article V, By-Laws of the RSC, RSC Coll.
33. C. W. Stiles to F. T. Gates, December 2, 1909, RSC Coll.
34. Article VIII, By-Laws of the RSC, RSC Coll.
35. Hackett MSS, chap. 3, p. 30.
36. Lewis W. Hackett, Notes taken from vol. 1 of the "Sourcebook for a History of the Rockefeller Foundation," collected by Catherine Lewirth, p. 539; both Hackett's notes and the "Sourcebook" are in the RF Archives.
37. Lewis W. Hackett, "Notes for IHD History," I, 76, RF Archives; Lewirth, "Sourcebook," p. 540.
38. Minutes, meeting of the Board of Directors, RSC, January 15, 1910, RSC Coll.
39. Lewirth, "Sourcebook," p. 541; address by Raymond B. Fosdick at a memorial meeting for Wickliffe Rose at the RI, February 25, 1932, in Hackett, "Notes," I, 71; Wickliffe Rose, *Report of the Administrative Secretary: Organization, Activities, and Results up to December 31, 1910*, RSC publication no. 3, (Washington: RSC, 1910), p. 3; Lewis W. Hackett's interview with Abraham Flexner, October 2, 1950, in Hackett, "Notes," I, 59.
40. From a typed, undated essay, probably written after Rose's retirement in 1928, entitled "Un matin à Olympia," RF Archives. The original passage states: "Les dialogues particulièrement avec la finesse de leur idéalisme m'ont entraîné dans un autre monde et dans une vie nouvelle. C'etait le commencement de ma vie intellectuelle."
41. Frederick Preston Rose, *My Father's People, 1650–1958: The Rose Family Through Three Hundred Years* (Atlanta: Preston Rose Co., n.d.); this is a printed, spiral-bound pamphlet without pagination, a copy of which is in the Wickliffe Rose Papers, RF Archives.
42. Hackett, "Notes," I, 76; Fosdick, *Rockefeller Foundation*, p. 12; graduation program from the University of Nashville, Peabody Normal College, May 28, 1890, RSC Coll.; Hackett MSS, chap. 3, pp. 30-34; *Nashville American*, July 6, 1910; Wickliffe Rose Correspondence, January-July 6, 1910, RSC Coll.
43. Quoted by Raymond Fosdick in an address at the RI, February 25, 1932, RF Archives.
44. Lewis W. Hackett's interview with Florence M. Read, November 22, 1950, in Hackett, "Notes," I, 458.
45. Wickliffe Rose – George Herbert Clarke correspondence, 1911–1918, RSC Coll. Clarke was on the faculty of the University of Tennessee. This particular poem evoked Rose's abiding interest in astronomy ("Dans lesquelles dansent / les etoiles en harmonie / Avec le grand choeur / de la nature.") Rose played a major role in the financing and construction of the 200-inch Hale telescope at Mt. Palomar.
46. David Starr Jordan and Ernest Alexander McGregor, "Description of a New Species of Trout (*Salmo Rosei*) from Culver Lake in the

High Sierras of California," *Proceedings of the Academy of Natural Scientists of Philadelphia*, 76 (1924), 19-22.

47. Lewirth, "Sourcebook," I, 541-542; Rose, "Work to Be Done," *Report of the Administrative Secretary.*

48. Rose, *"Work to Be Done,"* p. 3.

49. *Ibid.,* p. 4.

50. The twelve states referred to here as "Southern" are Virginia, North Carolina, South Carolina, Georgia, Florida, Mississippi, Alabama, Louisiana, Texas, Arkansas, Tennessee, and Kentucky.

51. RSC, publication no. 4, *State Systems of Public Health in Twelve Southern States* (Washington: RSC, 1911), *passim.*

52. Ibid., p. 11

53. Ibid., p. 22

54. Ibid., p. 66.

55. Ibid., p. 67.

56. Frederick Law Olmsted, *A Journey in the Back Country* (New York: Mason Brothers, 1860), pp. 342-343.

57. Article draft dated October 26, 1909, in the Walter Hines Page Papers.

58. Lewirth, "Sourcebook," I, 543.


## 6. Making the Idea Fashionable

1. Hackett MSS, chap. 3, p. 35; Harry Frank Farmer, "The Hookworm Eradication Program in the South," Ph.D. diss., University of Georgia, 1970, p. 78; "Hookworm Conference," *Journal of the American Medical Association*, 54 (January 29, 1910), 391-395.

2. Hackett MSS, chap. 3, p. 35; "The Conference for the Eradication of the Hookworm Disease," *Florida Health Notes*, 5 (February 1910), 25.

3. Charles W. Stiles to John A. Ferrell, February 3, 1939, RSC Coll.; RSC, publication no. 4, *State Systems of Public Health*, 14-17, 66.

4. Florida State Board of Health, *Twenty-first Annual Report: for 1909* (Jacksonville: Florida State Board of Health, 1910), pp. 21-24; "If He Only Knew," *Florida Health Notes*, 4 (March 1909), 44; Wickliffe Rose to Morgan Smith, May 12, 1910, RSC Coll. ("Quite a number of our men are making a journey to Florida to study the work which has been done in that state."); Wickliffe Rose to F. T. Gates, August 20, 1910, RSC Coll.

5. Lyman Abbott to William H. Welch, December 20, 1909, RSC Coll.; A. P. Bourland to Wickliffe Rose, February 25, 1910, RSC Coll.

6. Wickliffe Rose to Hon. J. M. Dickinson, June 22, 1910, RSC Coll.

7. Wickliffe Rose to Bailey K. Ashford, June 23, 1910, RSC Coll.

8. Unsigned Memorandum for the Secretary of War, February 7, 1910, RSC Coll.; Bailey K. Ashford to Hon. George Colton, January 18, 1910, RSC Coll.

9. Bailey K. Ashford, "Control and Eradication of Hookworm

Disease," n.d., MS in RSC Coll., covering letter accompanying the manuscript is dated August 18, 1912.

10. Wickliffe Rose to Bailey K. Ashford, June 23, 1910, RSC Coll.

11. Minutes, RSC, December 9, 1910, p. 1, RSC Coll.; Wickliffe Rose to Walter H. Page, November 14, 1910, RSC Coll. The RSC, no doubt at Gates's insistence, did not see fit to extend its work to include Puerto Rico. Rockefeller's original gift had been specifically earmarked for a campaign in the Southern states. Congress also turned a deaf ear to Ashford's and Colton's request for more funds to enlarge the work of the Anemia Commission; Bailey K. Ashford to Wickliffe Rose, October 24, 1911, August 18, 1912, and April 21, 1914, RSC Coll.

12. Edgar G. Murphy to Wickliffe Rose, February 9, 1910, RSC Coll. The emphasis is Murphy's.

13. Charles Wardell Stiles, "Some Recent Investigations into the Prevalence of Hookworm Disease Among Children," extract from an address delivered at the second annual meeting of the Child Conference for Research and Welfare, Worcester, Massachusetts, June/July 1910, p. 1, RSC Coll.

14. Allen W. Freeman to Wickliffe Rose, May 5, 1910, RSC Coll.

15. Greer Williams interview with Benjamin E. Washburn, September 30, 1963, Williams notes in RF Archives.

16. Charles W. Stiles to the residents of Wilmington, N.C., open letter dated April 5, 1914, RSC Coll.

17. Rose, *Report of the Administrative Secretary*, p. 13.

18. RSC, publication no. 9, *Fifth Annual Report for the Year 1914* (Washington: RSC, 1915), p. 21.

19. Quoted in Sullivan, *Our Times*, III, 327.

20. Washburn, *As I Recall*, p. 6.

21. *Arkansas Democrat*, February 18, 1913.

22. The quotation from the *Manufacturers' Record* was reprinted with favorable comments in the *New Orleans Daily Picayune*, the page of which was clipped and sent to Rose, without the date, by W. S. Leathers, on December 22, 1910, RSC Coll.

23. Ibid.

24. Hackett MSS, chap. 3, p. 27.

25. Josephus Daniels, *Editor in Politics* (Chapel Hill: University of North Carolina Press, 1941), p. 568. See also Ellsworth, "Theodore Roosevelt's Country Life Commission," pp. 167-168, 170-171.

26. Hackett MSS, chap. 3, p. 27.

27. Ibid., p. 27; Washburn, *As I Recall*, p. 6.

28. A. M. Wood to A. G. Fort, February 27, 1912, RSC Coll.

29. F. T. Gates to Wickliffe Rose, December 17, 1909, RSC Coll.

30. Hackett MSS, chap. 3, p. 27; Wickliffe Rose to Jerome Greene, December 23, 1913, RSC Coll.; W. M. Bumbry to Wickliffe Rose, May 30, 1910, RSC Coll.; A. P. Bourland to F. H. Peck, June 17, 1910, RSC Coll.; Ralph Steiner to Wickliffe Rose, April 10, 1911, RSC Coll.

31. Olin West to Wickliffe Rose, June 27, 1910, RSC Coll.

32. Reprinted in Sullivan, *Our Times*, III, 325.

33. E. E. Cummings, *i: Six Nonlectures* (Cambridge, Mass.: Harvard University Press, 1953), p. 29.

34. Mark Twain, *Letters from the Earth*, ed. Bernard De Voto (New York: Harper & Row, 1962), pp. 36-37.

35. Walter Hines Page, "The Hookworm and Civilization," *The World's Work*, 24 (September 1912), 504, 509.

36. Ibid., p. 509.

37. *Macon* (Georgia) *Telegraph*, September 25, 1912.

38. Lyman Abbott, "Hookworm Disease," *The Outlook*, November 13, 1909, p. 568.

39. Rose, *Report of the Administrative Secretary*, p. 5.

40. Wickliffe Rose to James Y. Joyner, January 10, 1910, RSC Coll.

41. C. W. Garrison to Wickliffe Rose, June 29, 1912, RSC Coll.; Hackett, "Notes," vol. 2, p. 795; Burrow, *Organized Medicine in the Progressive Era*, p. 27.

42. Rose, *Report of the Administrative Secretary*, pp. 5-6.

43. Ibid., p. 6. Louisiana did not appoint any inspectors until 1911.

44. Wickliffe Rose to W. H. Sanders, September 6, 1910, RSC Coll.

45. Ibid.

46. John A. Ferrell to Wickliffe Rose, June 6, 1910, RSC Coll.; Wickliffe Rose to W. S. Leathers, December 5, 1910, RSC Coll.

47. Wickliffe Rose to F. T. Gates, October 25, 1911, RSC Coll.

48. A. T. McCormack to Wickliffe Rose, December 22, 1911, August 9, 1912, February 7, 1913, RSC Coll.

49. Wickliffe Rose to C. W. Garrison, March 31, 1913, RSC Coll.

50. C. W. Garrison to A. T. McCormack, April 9, 1914, RSC Coll.

51. Wickliffe Rose to Bailey K. Ashford, December 15, 1910, RSC Coll.

52. Wickliffe Rose to Oscar Dowling, August 7, 1911, RSC Coll.; Wickliffe Rose to Morgan Smith, December 23, 1912, RSC Coll.; Minutes, RSC Executive Board, December 23, 1912, p. 3, RSC Coll.; Wickliffe Rose to W. F. Snow, September 11, 1911, RSC Coll.

53. Cassedy, "Germ of Laziness," p. 166.

54. Wickliffe Rose to Morgan Smith, May 12, 1910, RSC Coll.

55. Wickliffe Rose to J. A. Albright, May 18, 1910, RSC Coll.

56. Ibid.

57. Wickliffe Rose to S. D. Porter, September 24, 1912, RSC Coll.; Wickliffe Rose to R. H. Wilson, April 26, 1911, RSC Coll.

58. Wickliffe Rose to S. D. Porter, February 21, 1912, RSC Coll.; a typical letter to physicians is reprinted in "Exhibits" (chap. 4), RSC, publication no. 6, *Second Annual Report of the Rockefeller Sanitary Commission* (Washington: RSC, 1911), pp. 93-95.

59. Rose, *Report of the Administrative Secretary*, pp. 14, 15, appendicies 1-9 (for the maps of each of the nine participating states in 1910); W. S. Leathers to Wickliffe Rose, July 7, 1910, RSC Coll.; J. LaBruce Ward to Wickliffe Rose, November 22, 1910, RSC Coll.; John A. Ferrell to

Wickliffe Rose, April 23, 1910, May 19, 1910, August 3, 1910, RSC Coll.

60. Rose, *Report of the Administrative Secretary*, p. 15.

61. Ibid., p. 11.

62. These figures were computed from raw data included in Rose, *Report of the Administrative Secretary*, p. 25.

63. Ibid., p. 5.

64. S. D. Porter to J. C. Burdett, December 9, 1910, RSC Coll.

65. A. T. McCormack to the physicians of Muhlenberg County, Kentucky, July 2, 1914, RSC Coll.

66. Rose, *Report of the Administrative Secretary*, p. 25.

67. John A. Ferrell to Wickliffe Rose, April 23, 1910, RSC Coll.

68. Wickliffe Rose to Olin West, November 16, 1910, RSC Coll.

69. Rose, *Report of the Administrative Secretary*, p. 17.

70. *Bulletin of the Virginia Department of Health*, 2 (June 1910). On the title page, the word "retards" is misprinted as "regards."

71. Charles W. Stiles, *Soil Pollution as Cause of Ground-Itch, Hookworm Disease (Ground-Itch Anemia), and Dirt-Eating: A Circular for Use in Schools*, RSC publication no. 1 (Washington: RSC, 1910), p. 4. The emphasis is Stiles's.

72. Ibid., p. 6.

73. Rose, *Report of the Administrative Secretary*, p. 21.

74. S. N. Carven to S. H. Jacobs, December 1, 1912, RSC Coll.

75. Rose, *Report of the Administrative Secretary*, p. 21.

76. Daniels, *Editor in Politics*, pp. 568-569; RSC, publication no. 6, *Second Annual Report*, p. 108; Rose, *Report of the Administrative Secretary*, p. 28.

77. Huntsville, Alabama, *Weekly Mercury*, December 4, 1912.

78. Ibid.

79. Wickliffe Rose to W. H. Page, October 29, 1910, RSC Coll.

80. Wickliffe Rose to A. W. Freeman, September 15, 1910, RSC Coll.

81. Wickliffe Rose to A. W. Freeman, March 3, 1911, RSC Coll.

82. Rose, *Report of the Administrative Secretary*, p. 28.

83. A. G. Fort to Wickliffe Rose, August 20, 1910, RSC Coll.; Wickliffe Rose to A. G. Fort, September 30, 1911, RSC Coll.; Morgan Smith to Wickliffe Rose, August 28, 1911, RSC Coll.; Wickliffe Rose to Morgan Smith, August 30, 1911, RSC Coll.; W. S. Leathers to Wickliffe Rose, January 19, 1912, RSC Coll.; W. S. Leathers to Wickliffe Rose, November 25, 1910, RSC Coll.; James K. Vardaman to W. S. Leathers, July 25, 1913, RSC Coll.; Earl Brewer to W. S. Leathers, July 28, 1913, RSC Coll.

## 7. *The Days of Galilee*

1. Rose, *Report of the Administrative Secretary*, p. 26.

2. Wickliffe Rose to F. T. Gates, March 6, 1911, RSC Coll.

3. RSC, publication no. 6, *Second Annual Report*, p. 9.

4. Compiled from data taken from Rose, *Report of the Administra-*

*tive Secretary*, p. 14, and from RSC, publication no. 6, *Second Annual Report*, p. 8.

5. RSC, publication no. 6, *Second Annual Report*, p. 8; S. D. Porter to Wickliffe Rose, January 17, 1911, RSC Coll.

6. A. W. Freeman to Wickliffe Rose, March 4, 1911, April 15, 1911, RSC Coll.

7. S. D. Porter to Wickliffe Rose, January 17, 1911, January 19, 1911, RSC Coll.

8. Charles Wardell Stiles, "Hospital Relief for the Country," *Public Health Reports*, 28 (1913), 208-212; *Annual Report, Commissioner of Health of Virginia, Ending September 30, 1911* (Richmond: Virginia State Board of Health, 1911), pp. 22-23; *Biennial Report of the Louisiana State Board of Health to the General Assembly of the State of Louisiana, 1910–1911* (New Orleans: Louisiana State Board of Health, 1912), pp. 27-47; John Duffy, ed., *The Rudolph Matas History of Medicine in Louisiana*, 2 vols. (Baton Rouge: Louisiana State University Press, 1958–1962), II, 483-485.

9. A. T. McCormack to Wickliffe Rose, August 9, 1912, RSC Coll.

10. C. W. Garrison to Wickliffe Rose, November 19, 1911, RSC Coll. The poem is included in a brochure from the Arkansas Federation of Women's Clubs, "Baby Health Contest," dated October 26, 1913, a copy of which is in the RSC Coll.

11. Flannery O'Connor, "The Crop," in *The Complete Stories of Flannery O'Connor* (New York: Farrar, Straus and Giroux, 1971), pp. 34-35. "The Crop" was written before February 1946 but was first published in *Mademoiselle*, 72 (April 1971).

12. M. H. Boerner to Wickliffe Rose, November 17, 1913, RSC Coll.

13. J. A. Ferrell to Wickliffe Rose, December 1, 1911, RSC Coll.; Wickliffe Rose to A. W. Freeman, December 26, 1911, RSC Coll.; Wickliffe Rose to A. G. Fort, September 4, 1912, RSC Coll.; A. T. McCormack to Wickliffe Rose, July 11, 1913, RSC Col.; G. B. Adams to J. A. Ferrell, August 27, 1914, RSC Coll.

14. John C. Culley to Wickliffe Rose, March 7, 1911, RSC Coll.

15. W. S. Leathers to A. P. Bourland, June 28, 1910, RSC Coll.; W. S. Leathers, response to an RF inquiry, February 4, 1939, RSC Coll.; Wickliffe Rose to F. T. Gates, March 8, 1911, RSC Coll.

16. Hackett MSS, chap. 3, p. 12.

17. John C. Culley, response to an RF inquiry, May 29, 1939, RSC Coll.

18. W. S. Leathers to Wickliffe Rose, December 7, 1910, RSC Coll.; W. S. Leathers MS, "Dispensary Work in Mississippi," n.d., p. 2, RSC Coll.; W. S. Leathers, "Dispensary Work in Mississippi," *Southern Medical Journal*, 5 (February 1912).

19. Rose, *Report of the Administrative Secretary*, p. 19.

20. Wickliffe Rose to W. S. Leathers, January 26, 1911, RSC Coll.

21. Wickliffe Rose to Bailey K. Ashford, August 17, 1911, RSC Coll.; Leathers MS, "Dispensary Work in Mississippi," p. 5; Wickliffe Rose to

F. T. Gates, May 31, 1911, RSC Coll.; Joseph Blotner, *Faulkner: A Biography*, 2 vols. (New York: Random House, 1974), pp. 664, 681-683. William Faulkner blamed Dr. Culley for the death of his infant daughter, Alabama, in 1931.

22. RSC, publication no. 6, *Second Annual Report*, p. 18.

23. Ibid., p. 103.

24. Ibid., p. 21. Compare this description of Southern farm families on their way to a dispensary with the following passage, written by Nathan Cole, on the response of Connecticut farmers to the news that George Whitefield was to preach in nearby Middletown on October 23, 1740. "On high land I saw a cloud of fog rising. I first thought it came from the great river, but as I came nearer the road I heard a noise of horses' feet coming down the road, and this cloud was a cloud of dust made by the horses' feet . . . as I drew nearer it seemed like a steady stream of horses and their riders . . . and when we got to Middletown old meeting house, there was a great multitude, it was said to be 3 or 4,000 of people, assembled together . . . I turned and looked towards the Great River and saw the ferry boats running swift backward and forward bringing over loads of people." From Alan Heimert and Perry Miller, eds., *The Great Awakening* (Indianapolis: Bobbs-Merrill, 1967), pp. 185-186.

25. Washburn, *As I Recall*, pp. 12-14.

26. Minutes, RSC Executive Committee, April 4, 1913, p. 1, RSC Coll.

27. J. F. Orr to W. W. Dinsmore, September 9, 1913, RSC Coll.

28. W. W. Richmond to A. T. McCormack, December 7, 1912, RSC Coll.

29. A. T. McCormack to Wickliffe Rose, September 22, 1913, RSC Coll. See also J. S. Lock to A. T. McCormack, October 28, 1913, RSC Coll.

30. This percentage is based on a total of 694,494; see RSC, publication no. 9, *Fifth Annual Report*, p. 43.

31. Olin West to John A. Ferrell, September 23, 1913, RSC Coll.; Allen W. Freeman to Wickliffe Rose, February 7, 1914, RSC Coll.; RSC, publication no. 8, *Fourth Annual Report for the Year 1913* (Washington: RSC, 1914), p. 23.

32. C. W. Stiles to Wickliffe Rose, August 15, 1912, RSC Coll.

33. Wickliffe Rose to C. W. Stiles, August 24, 1912, RSC Coll.

34. John A. Ferrell, *Hookworm Disease: Its Ravages, Prevention and Cure* (Washington: RSC, 1915), pp. 24-25.

35. Ibid., p. 25.

36. Charles W. Stiles to Wickliffe Rose, July 9, 1911, RSC Coll.

37. Ibid.

38. See A. W. Wood to A. G. Fort, February 23, 1914, RSC Coll.

39. Charles W. Stiles to Wickliffe Rose, July 9, 1911, RSC Coll.; John A. Ferrell to Wickliffe Rose, August 9, 1911, RSC Coll.

40. Charles W. Stiles to Wickliffe Rose, August 28, 1912, RSC Coll.; RSC, publication no. 7, *Third Annual Report* (Washington: RSC, 1912), p. 5.

41. Stiles's annual salary from the Sanitary Commission was $2,500. Using Rose's annual salary of $7,500 for full-time work as an index (in theory, at least, the two occupied separate and equal positions in the Commission's hierarchy), Stiles was giving approximately one-third of his time to the Commission.

42. RSC, publication no. 5, *Second Annual Report*, pp. 24-25; C. W. Stiles to Wickliffe Rose, October 7, 1911, RSC Coll.

43. RSC, publication no. 9, *Fifth Annual Report*, pp. 13-14. Rose miscalculated the sanitary index at 8 working with the figures in this example.

44. Charles Wardell Stiles, *First Annual Report of the Scientific Secretary for the Year Ending January 25, 1911*, RSC, publication no. 2 (Washington: RSC, 1911, pp. 12-17.

45. C. W. Stiles to Wickliffe Rose, June 7, 1915, RSC Coll.

46. John A. Ferrell to C. W. Garrison, August 30, 1913, RSC Coll.

47. J. LaB. Ward to Wickliffe Rose, February 28, 1913, RSC Coll.; see also Sidney Porter to Wickliffe Rose, November 2, 1911, RSC Coll.; A. T. McCormack to John A. Ferrell, August 18, 1915, RSC Coll.; M. H. Boerner to John A. Ferrell, January 30, 1914, RSC Coll.

48. Blanche Rogers to the RI, November 19, 1914, RSC Coll.

49. Wickliffe Rose to C. W. Garrison, November 8, 1912, RSC Coll.

50. John A. Ferrell to C. T. Young, April 13, 1914, RSC Coll.

51. Stiles, *Hookworm Disease in its Relation to the Negro*, p. 4.

52. Ibid., p. 6.

53. Marion Hamilton Carter, "The Vampire of the South," *McClure's Magazine*, 33 (October 1909), 631.

54. Dr. Charles T. Nesbitt, "The Health Menace of Alien Races," *The World's Work*, 28 (November 1913), 74-75. An article by Allen Tullos, "The Great Hookworm Crusade," *Southern Exposure*, 6 (Summer 1978), 40-49, brought the Carter and Nesbitt articles to my attention. For an excellent discussion of Southern "racial medicine" in the progressive era, see the early chapters of James H. Jones, *Bad Blood: The Tuskegee Syphilis Experiment* (New York: The Free Press, 1981), which I was fortunately permitted to read in galley proof as this study was being prepared for print.

55. Wickliffe Rose to W. W. Dinsmore, June 17, 1912, RSC Coll.

56. John A. Ferrell to Wickliffe Rose, August 8, 1910, RSC Coll.

57. Wickliffe Rose to W. W. Dinsmore, June 17, 1912, RSC Coll.

58. "Open Letter from H. H. Howard, M.D., to the Leading Farmers and Planters of Winston County, Mississippi," attached to a letter from W. S. Leathers to Wickliffe Rose, June 26, 1912, RSC Coll.

59. Wickliffe Rose to A. W. Freeman, November 28, 1911, RSC Coll.

60. C. W. Garrison to Wickliffe Rose, June 7, 1913, RSC Coll.

61. C. W. Garrison to John A. Ferrell, April 27, 1914, RSC Coll.

62. John A. Ferrell to Wickliffe Rose, February 13, 1911, RSC Coll.; Wickliffe Rose to W. W. Dinsmore, July 22, 1913, RSC Coll.

63. Wickliffe Rose to W. S. Leathers, December 5, 1912, RSC Coll.

## 8. "Henceforth Thy Field Is the World"

1. Frederick T. Gates to John D. Rockefeller, June 3, 1905, RF Archives. See also Fosdick, *Rockefeller Foundation*, chaps. 1, 2; Gates, *Chapters in My Life*, pp. 207-209.

2. John D. Rockefeller, Jr., to John D. Rockefeller, December 31, 1906, RF Archives.

3. Fosdick, *Rockefeller Foundation*, p. 16.

4. Ibid., p. 16; *The New York Times*, March 3, 1910.

5. Jerome D. Greene, "Statement on the Proposed Incorporation of The Rockefeller Foundation," March 15, 1912, submitted as part of Report no. 529 to the United States House of Representatives, April 11, 1912; Hearing before the Committee on the District of Columbia, United States Senate, on the bill S. 6888 to incorporate The Rockefeller Foundation, March 11, 1910; see Fosdick, *Rockefeller Foundation*, pp. 16-17.

6. Collier and Horowitz, *The Rockefellers*, p. 64.

7. Fosdick, *Rockefeller Foundation*, p. 18.

8. *New York American*, March 4, 1910.

9. Henry F. Pringle, *The Life and Times of William Howard Taft*, 2 vols. (New York: Farrar & Rinehart, 1932), II, 662-663.

10. Ibid., p. 663.

11. United States Commission on Industrial Relations, 1913–1915, *Final Report*, 11 vols. (Washington: Government Printing Office, 1916), IX, 8814.

12. Quoted in Collier and Horowitz, *The Rockefellers*, p. 3.

13. It will be remembered that Gates had become a Congregationalist. Much of the force of Gladden's objection was lost when it was later learned that the Board of Missions of the Congregational Church had solicited the gift. See Gates, *Chapters in My Life*, pp. 198-205; Nevins, *Study in Power*, II, 345-347. For Gladden's side of the story, see Washington Gladden, *Recollections* (Boston: Houghton Mifflin, 1909).

14. Nevins, *Study in Power*, II, 365-368; Nevins, *John D. Rockefeller*, II, 508-511.

15. The dissolution of Standard Oil did not, however, constitute a financial blow to Rockefeller. When shares of stock in the various constituent companies were traded on Wall Street for the first time, the value of the stocks rose $200 million in five months. Rockefeller personally owned (and was allowed to retain, under the terms of the court order) 24.85 percent of the stock in the thirty-nine companies; see Collier and Horowitz, *The Rockefellers*, p. 59.

16. Lewirth, "Sourcebook," I, 529-530.

17. Jerome Greene-Wickliffe Rose Correspondence, May 23 and May 27, 1912, RSC Coll.

18. The original trustees of the Rockefeller Foundation, named in the act of incorporation, were Rockefeller, Sr. (who never attended a meeting); Rockefeller, Jr.; Gates; Harry Pratt Judson, president of the University of Chicago; Flexner; Murphy; Greene; Rose; and Charles O.

Heydt, the younger Rockefeller's private secretary. A short time later, two more men were added: Charles W. Eliot, president of Harvard University, and A. Barton Hepburn, president of the Rockefeller-controlled Chase National Bank. See Fosdick, *Rockefeller Foundation,* p.21.

19. First christened the International Health Commission, it was renamed the International Health Board in 1916. In 1927, it was renamed again, this time as the International Health Division. Its activities were brought to a close, and it passed out of legal existence, in 1951. Since this study is interested only insofar as it is an outgrowth of the Sanitary Commission and is concerned with events before 1916, when the first change of names occurred, the organization will hereafter in this chapter be referred to as the International Health Commission.

20. "Resolutions Establishing the International Health Commission" RF Archives.

21. Gates, *Chapters in My Life,* p. 225.

22. Ibid., p. 225; Hackett MSS, chap. 4, p. 4.

23. RSC, publication no. 6, *Hookworm Infection in Foreign Countries* (Washington: RSC, 1911), pp. 3-4.

24. The original International Health Commission included Rockefeller, Jr., chairman; Rose, director; Greene, recording secretary; Eliot; Welch; Gates; Page; Houston (then in Woodrow Wilson's cabinet as Secretary of Agriculture); William Crawford Gorgas, of yellow fever fame; Flexner; Murphy; and Heydt.

25. Hackett MSS, chap. 4, p. 57.

26. This quotation is from a journal kept by Rose on his trip to England, RF Archives.

27. Ibid.

28. Ibid., see also RF, *Annual Report, 1913-14* (New York: RF, 1915), pp.43-46.

29. RF, *Annual Report, 1913-14,* pp. 46-47, 72; Hackett, "Notes," III, 1443.

30. Hackett, "Notes," III, 1443.

31. Ibid., pp. 1443-1445; Victor Heiser, *An American Doctor's Odyssey: Adventures in Forty-five Countries* (New York: W. W. Norton, 1936), p. 266; RF, *Annual Report, 1913-14,* pp. 47-52.

32. John A. Ferrell's desk book, entry dated January 19, 1914, RF Archives.

33. Wickliffe Rose to John A. Ferrell, February 26, 1914, RSC Coll; see also Minutes, RSC annual meeting, January 1914, RSC Coll.

34. Wickliffe Rose to John A. Ferrell, February 26, 1914, RSC Coll.

35. Ferrell's recollections of the meeting of the executive committee of the IHC are contained in the transcription of an interview with him conducted in 1939. The transcription, dated April 19 (no year), was submitted in connection with the compilation of data by Lewirth and is in the RF Archives.

36. Lewis Hackett's interview with W. P. Jacocks, April 25 and 26, 1951, RF Archives; Lewis Hackett's interview with John A. Ferrell,

April 25, 1951, RF Archives; the Rockefellers' interest in Colorado Fuel and Iron is extensively documented in the United States Commission on Industrial Relations, *Final Report*, VIII, 7763; the correspondence between Rockefeller, Jr. and Bowers is in IX, 8411-8449. For a thorough discussion of the events in Colorado, see George S. McGovern and Leonard F. Guttridge, *The Great Coalfield War* (Boston: Houghton Mifflin, 1972), and Graham Adams, Jr., *The Age of Industrial Violence, 1910-1915* (New York: Columbia University Press, 1966).

37. The events surrounding the Ludlow Massacre have been brought up in the context of this study for the purpose of demonstrating their retarding impact on the early efforts of the Rockefeller Foundation. For full accounts of the incident, see McGovern and Guttridge, *The Great Coalfield War;* Adams, *Industrial Violence;* and James Weinstein, *The Corporate Ideal in the Liberal State, 1900-1918* (Boston: Beacon Press, 1968), chap. 7.

38. Collier and Horowitz, *The Rockefellers*, p. 118.

39. Ibid., pp. 120-122; RF, *Annual Report, 1913-14*, pp. 16-23.

40. Ferrell remembered that in the spring of 1914, the Rockefeller offices at 26 Broadway were busy "preparing data for the use of those called by the commission to submit testimony." See the Ferrell transcription, April 19, 193(9), RF Archives.

41. Weinstein, *The Corporate Ideal in the Liberal State*, p. 205.

42. Charles V. Chapin, *A Report on State Public Health Work Based on a Survey of State Boards of Health* (Chicago: American Medical Association, 1915), p. 106.

43. Ibid., p. 107.

44. John A. Ferrell to J. LaB. Ward, August 1, 1913, RSC Coll.

45. Allen Freeman to Wickliffe Rose, September 4, 1914, RSC Coll.

46. Wickliffe Rose to Allen Freeman, September 8, 1914, RSC Coll.

47. A. T. McCormack to John A. Ferrell, June 3, 1914, RSC Coll.

48. Jerome Greene to John D. Rockefeller, Jr., August 29, 1914, RSC Coll.

49. Frederick T. Gates to Wickliffe Rose, August 21, 1914, RSC Coll., the emphasis is Gates's.

50. Lewis W. Hackett's interview with Raymond Fosdick, May 1951, RF Archives.

51. Frederick T. Gates to John D. Rockefeller, August 19, 1914, RSC Coll.

52. John D. Rockefeller to the members of the RSC, August 12, 1914, RSC Coll.

53. Wickliffe Rose, "Recommendation of Plan for Closing the Work of the Rockefeller Sanitary Commission in the Southern States," appended to the minutes of the meeting of the RSC executive committee, September 25, 1914, RSC Coll.

54. Lewirth, "Sourcebook," I, 564.

55. Ferrell transcription, April 19, 193(9), RF Archives.

56. Frederick T. Gates, "Philanthropy and Civilization," paper presented to the RF trustees, 1923, RF Archives.

57. Gates, *Chapters in My Life*, p. 186.

58. Frederick T. Gates to Charles W. Eliot, November 1, 1910, RF Archives.

59. John A. Ferrell, "What the Rockefeller Sanitary Commission Can Do to Build up County Health Work," *Bulletin of the North Carolina State Board of Health,* 27 (August 1912), 171-174.

60. Ibid., p. 174.

61. E. Richard Brown, *Rockefeller Medicine Men: Medicine and Capitalism in America* (Berkeley: University of California Press, 1979).

62. Brown, *Rockefeller Medicine Men,* p. 117.

63. Ibid., p. 116.

64. Howard S. Berliner, "Philanthropic Foundations and Scientific Medicine," Sc.D. dissertation, The Johns Hopkins University, 1977, chap. 2; Merle Curti, *American Philanthropy Abroad* (New Brunswick: Rutgers University Press, 1963); Ernest R. May, "Missionary and World Power: America's Destiny in the Twentieth Century," in *American Civilization: A Portrait from the Twentieth Century,* ed. Daniel Boorstin (New York: McGraw-Hill, 1972).

65. Frederick T. Gates, "The Letter on Missions," n.d., RF Archives; "Jerome Davis Greene," RF, *Confidential Report,* no. 197, April 1959, RF Archives; RF, *Annual Report, 1913-14,* pp. 29-34.

66. Richard Hofstadter, *Social Darwinism in American Thought,* rev. ed. (Boston: Beacon Press, 1955); Charles Coulston Gillispie, *Genesis and Geology: The Impact of Scientific Discoveries Upon Religious Beliefs in the Decades Before Darwin* (Cambridge, Mass.: Harvard University Press, 1951).

67. Berliner, "Philanthropic Foundations," p. 109.

68. Ibid., p. 122.

69. Hookworm disease was certainly a function of rural poverty, and more recent investigation has explored the relationship between nutrition and susceptibility.

70. Charles Rosenberg has suggested an evangelical basis for the early public health programs in New York in the 1840s in his *No Other Gods,* chap. 6, "Piety and Social Action: Origins of the American Public Health Movement."

71. Even the parasite's scientific names, when spoken, might invoke this association, at least in the mind of a layman like Gates: *Uncinaria* (un-sin = "sin no more") and *Necator* (sin = death). Edgar Allen Poe had used the worm as a symbol of decay, corruption, and the power of evil in *The Conqueror Worm* (1843).

72. Paul E. Johnson, *A Shopkeeper's Millennium: Society and Revivals in Rochester, New York, 1815-1837* (New York: Hill and Wang, 1978), p. 135.

*Epilogue*

1. RF, IHB, *Annual Report for 1926* (New York: RF, 1927), p. 84.

2. Stiles, "Early History," p. 305.

3. Lewirth, "Sourcebook," I, 558.

4. Ibid.

5. Charles Wardell Stiles, "Is It Fair to Say That Hookworm Disease

Has Almost Disappeared from the United States?," *Science,* 77 (March 3, 1933), 237-239; C. W. Stiles to J. A. Ferrell, February 3, 1939, RSC Coll.

6. Lewirth, "Sourcebook," I, 560-562.

7. Ibid., p. 562.

8. Donald L. Augustine and Wilson G. Smillie, "The Relation of the Types of Soil in Alabama to the Distribution of Hookworm Disease," *American Journal of Hygiene,* 6, March Supplement (March 1926), 51-52.

9. Norman R. Stoll, "This Wormy World," *Journal of Parasitology,* 33 (February 1933), 8.

10. Paul C. Beaver, address to the Conference of the World Association for the Advancement of Parasitology, meeting in Philadelphia in September 1965, summarized in a *Science Service* release, September 8, 1965, RSC Coll.

11. One is surprised that Stiles, who was always a thorn in the sides of the Rockefeller administrators, was able to work so long and in such apparent harmony within the largest bureaucracy of them all, the federal government.

12. C. L. Pridgen to J. A. Ferrell, April 3, 1914, RSC Coll.

13. RSC, publication no. 9, *Fifth Annual Report,* pp. 23-24. The final figures for all anti-hookworm work in the Southern states – number of people examined, treatments dispensed, and privies constructed – would have to include the six months' worth of work carried out under the auspices of the IHC. These results may be found in RF, IHC, *Annual Report: 1915* (New York: RF, 1916). Only statistics that reflect work done exclusively under the direction of the RSC have been included in this summary of accomplishments.

14. Lewis W. Hackett's interview with John A. Ferrell, November 3, 1950, in Hackett, "Notes," I, 293.

15. Ibid.

16. RF, IHC, *Annual Report: 1915,* pp. 219-221; Brown, *Basic Clinical Parasitology,* p. 128; Beeson and McDermott, *Textbook of Medicine,* p. 526.

17. John D. Rockefeller to the members of the original board of directors of the RSC, October 26, 1909, RSC Coll.

18. Clark, *The Emerging South,* p. 27.

19. RSC, publication no. 9, *Fifth Annual Report,* pp. 11-12.

20. Francis Arthur Bell, in response to a RF questionnaire, February 10, 1939, RF Archives.

21. RSC, publication no. 9, *Fifth Annual Report,* pp. 12-13.

22. Ibid., pp. 13-14.

23. Ibid., p. 46.

24. Ibid., p. 20. Earlier it was noted that there were 19,981 licensed physicians in the South. This lower figure represented the number in the original nine states in 1910; the higher figure cited in this paragraph denotes the number in eleven states four years later.

25. Leila (Georgia) School Program, March 20, 1914, RSC Coll.

26. Only 75 of Texas' 249 counties, all located in the eastern part of the state, were counted in the infected zone.

27. A. G. Fort to Wickliffe Rose, June 21, 1913, RSC Coll.

28. Wickliffe Rose to A. G. Fort, June 23, 1913, RSC Coll.

29. See RF, IHC, *Annual Report: 1915.*

30. United States Bureau of Education, Bulletin, no. 20, *The Rural School and Hookworm Disease* (Washington: Government Printing Office, 1914); RSC, publication no. 9, *Fifth Annual Report,* pp. 22-23.

31. RSC, publication no. 9, *Fifth Annual Report,* pp. 42-43.

32. Ibid., p. 50.

33. W. S. Rankin to Wickliffe Rose, December 16, 1911, RSC Coll.

34. Greer Williams' interview with W. S. Rankin, September 30, 1963, RF Archives.

35. Woodward, *Origins of the New South,* p. 426.

36. RSC, publication no. 9, *Fifth Annual Report,* p. 26.

37. William H. Glasson, "The Rockefeller Commission's Campaign Against the Hookworm," *The South Atlantic Quarterly,* 10 (April 1911), p. 148.

38. RSC, publication no. 9, *Fifth Annual Report,* pp. 26-27.

39. Wickliffe Rose to F. T. Gates, May 16, 1911, RSC Coll.; Wickliffe Rose to F. T. Gates, November 22, 1911, RSC Coll.; Wickliffe Rose to F. T. Gates, November 22, 1911, RSC Coll.; W. S. Rankin to Wickliffe Rose, March 25, 1911, RSC Coll.; Allen W. Freeman, "Rural Health Organization in the United States: Past, Present, and Future," *Southern Medical Journal,* 27 (June 1934), 518; John A. Ferrell and Pauline A. Mead, "History of County Health Organizations in the United States, 1908-1933," United States Public Health Service, *Bulletin,* no. 222 (March 1936); RSC, publication no. 9, *Fifth Annual Report,* pp. 48-49.

# A Note
# on the Sources

There has been no previous monograph on the Rockefeller Sanitary Commission, no doubt in large part because until 1974 its records were unavailable to scholars. The student of the Commission, unless hand-picked and employed by the Rockefeller Foundation, was forced to rely on its nine publications: publication no. 1, Charles Wardell Stiles, *Soil Pollution as Cause of Ground-Itch, Hookworm Disease (Ground-Itch Anemia), and Dirt Eating: A Circular for Use in Schools* (Washington: RSC, 1910); publication no. 2, *First Annual Report of the Scientific Secretary for the Year Ending January 25, 1911* (Washington: RSC, 1911); publication no. 3, *Report of the Administrative Secretary: Organization, Activities, and Results up to December 31, 1910* (Washington: RSC, 1911); publication no. 4, *State Systems of Public Health in Twelve Southern States* (Washington: RSC, 1911); publication no. 5, *Second Annual Report* (Washington: RSC, 1911); publication no. 6, *Hookworm Infection in Foreign Countries* (Washington: RSC, 1911); publication no. 7, *Third Annual Report* (Washington: RSC, 1912); publication no. 8, *Fourth Annual Report for the Year 1913* (Washington: RSC, 1914); publication no. 9, *Fifth Annual Report for the Year 1914* (Washington: RSC, 1915). In addition, results of Rockefeller-sponsored work in the South can be found in the International Health Commission's sections of The Rockefeller Foundation, *Annual Report: 1913-14* (New York: RF, 1915), and The Rockefeller Foundation, *Annual Report: 1915* (New York: RF, 1916). Each annual report is more than a perfunctory recitation of the previous year's accomplishments. Each does include, as one might expect, data from the participating states in the form of tables, charts, graphs, and maps; but each also contains a wealth of additional information of a less quantitative nature such as letters from field workers and former hookworm victims, personal observations, and photographs. Another indispensable resource is The Rockefeller Foundation, International Health Board, publication no. 11, *Bibliography of Hookworm Disease* (New York: RF, 1922), a cross-referenced list of virtually every journal article and monograph on the subject before 1922. Its introduction provides a good, brief summary of the history of hookworm disease.

Since 1974, the Commission's papers have been open for research. They form the evidentiary base for much of this study. The archival materials on the Sanitary Commission encompass six shelf feet and three bound volumes of minutes, administrative records, financial data, reports from the sanitary workers in the field, and files of correspondence. Apparently no one at the Commission's headquarters ever threw anything away. Every aspect of its activities is represented.

The Sanitary Commission papers are housed at the Rockefeller Archive Center, located on the Rockefeller estate outside Tarrytown, New York. Also kept here are the records of the other Rockefeller philanthropic organizations, including the General Education Board, the Rockefeller Institute (now Rockefeller University), and the Rockefeller Family and Associates collection.

The papers of most of the key figures associated with the work of the Sanitary Commission are also deposited at the Rockefeller Archive Center. The personal papers of John D. Rockefeller and John D. Rockefeller, Jr., are here and may be studied on application to the archivist. The Frederick T. Gates collection takes up two shelf feet and includes correspondence with his employer, unpublished essays, and the fascinating and valuable "Autobiography," written in 1928 and published under the title *Chapters in My Life* (New York: Free Press, 1977). One may also inspect the papers of Wallace Buttrick (107 items and two volumes), John A. Ferrell (approximately 400 items), and Wickliffe Rose (a meager one shelf foot).

Unfortunately, Stiles did not systematically save his personal papers. Some are at the Rockefeller Archive Center; others at the Academy of Natural Sciences in Philadelphia; still others in the Library of Congress. What personal papers do exist shed little light on either the career or the private life of this important and complicated figure. One must fall back on his scientific publications (numerous) and the few "authorized" biographical sketches. These include Frank G. Brooks, "Charles Wardell Stiles: Intrepid Scientist," *Bios*, 18 (1947), 139-169; Mark Sullivan, *Our Times:*

*The United States, 1900-1925,* 6 vols. (New York: Charles
Scribner's Sons, 1930), III, 299-303; Benjamin Schwartz, "A Brief
Resumé of Dr. Stiles' Contributions to Parasitology," *Journal of
Parasitology,* 19 (June 1933), 257-261; Stiles's own "Early
History, in Part Esoteric, of the Hookworm (Uncinariasis) Cam-
paign in Our Southern States," *Journal of Parasitology,* 25
(August 1939), 283-308; and James H. Cassedy's brief sketch,
"Charles Wardell Stiles," in *DSB,* XIII (1976), 62-63.

Up until 1974, each secondary work on the Rockefellers and
their empire fell into one of two categories: "house histories"
based on archival material made available to carefully chosen
scholars working for the Foundation, or critical studies whose
authors were denied access to the more than 20 million pieces of
paper making up the Rockefeller Collection and forced to make do
with newspaper articles, public documents, Foundation publications, and secondary works. I have relied heavily on seven of
these approved histories – six published and one in manuscript.
Allan Nevin's biography, *John D. Rockefeller: The Heroic Age of
American Enterprise,* 2 vols. (New York: Charles Scribner's Sons,
1940), represented the culmination of a twenty-year search for
the appropriate biographer. Among those considered before the
job was offered to Nevins were Emil Ludwig (who was bored by
the elder Rockefeller, in whom he detected little resemblance to
Napoleon) and Winston Churchill (who asked for too much
money). Nevins later revised his book to take advantage of some
documents that had come to light after the first version was in
print. The second edition was called *John D. Rockefeller: A Study
in Power,* 2 vols. (New York: Charles Scribner's Sons, 1953). In
neither edition (less so in the second) will the reader find
Rockefeller seriously taken to task for violations of law or abuses
of power during his long struggle to build and protect Standard
Oil. Nevins viewed the concentration of capital at the end of the
nineteenth century as inevitable and good. He also implied that
responsible empire-builders like Rockefeller helped the United
States to avoid the two twentieth-century alternatives of fascism
and communism. Raymond Fosdick, unlike Nevins, made no
claims to objectivity. He was a life-long friend of the younger
Rockefeller as well as a president of the Rockefeller Foundation.
It is not at all surprising, then, to discover that his *John D.
Rockefeller, Jr.: A Portrait* (New York: Harper & Brothers, 1956)
conceals the blemishes and highlights the strong features of its
subject. The Ludlow tragedy, for example, becomes in Fosdick's
telling just one of the trials life contrived to strew in the younger

Rockefeller's path, and which he managed to overcome in the process of forging his exemplary character. However flagrant the biases or however unfashionable the points of view expressed in Fosdick's and Nevin's biographies, they still stand as unrivaled sources of detailed information. The same can be said of Fosdick's two monographs cited in the fourth chapter of this study: *The Story of the Rockefeller Foundation* (New York: Harper & Brothers, 1952), and *Adventure in Giving: The Story of the General Education Board, a Foundation Established by John D. Rockefeller* (New York: Harper & Row, 1962). The latter is based on an unfinished manuscript by Henry F. and Katherine Douglas Pringle. These books, along with another authorized history, George Corner's *A History of the Rockefeller Institute, 1901-1953: Origins and Growth* (New York: RI Press, 1964), will save the serious student of the early Rockefeller philanthropies — enthusiast, critic, and disinterested scholar alike — much repetitious work in the documents.

Sometimes in the mid-1930s, Catherine Lewirth, of the Foundation's staff, began to compile information to be used in a history of the Rockefeller Foundation. Lewirth not only put random documents together in narrative form but also corresponded extensively with former employees. The Pringles and Fosdick drew heavily on the several volumes of her "Sourcebook," as did Lewis W. Hackett, a retired Foundation public health physician, commissioned to write a history of the International Health Division (a.k.a. Commission and Board). Before his death in 1962, Hackett had amassed on his own 1,500 pages of typewritten notes, many more pages of notes in his own hand, and nine chapters of a first draft. This study rests in part on Hackett's labors, especially on his notes, his correspondence and interviews with former associates, and the third and fourth chapters of his manuscript. Greer Williams was hired by the Foundation to take over and complete Hackett's history. He in turn built up a file of his own notes, interviews, and correspondence, all of which are housed, with Hackett's research materials, at the Rockefeller Archive Center. Williams's book, *The Plague Killers* (New York: Charles Scribner's Sons, 1969), a fast-paced thriller in *The Microbe Hunters* tradition, does not reflect the layers of painstaking work that went into its creation.

Peter Collier's and David Horowitz's *The Rockefellers: An American Dynasty* (New York: Holt, Rinehart and Winston, 1976) represented a departure in the historiography of Rockefeller studies. Collier and Horowitz were given access to the materials of the Rockefeller Archives through the intercession of several members of the fourth generation of Rockefellers (referred to generically as "The Cousins" in the book). Employees of the Foundation were instructed to cooperate in Collier's and Horowitz's investigation and to make available to them all records heretofore reserved for the eyes of the house historians only. Since they were neither beholden to the Foundation nor especially predisposed to admire the family, their book is at once well researched and irreverent. The fact that it covers four generations in one volume, however, precludes its moving on the same level of detail found in the Nevins, Fosdick, and Corner studies.

Three recent journal articles take up the subject of the Sanitary Commission. Mary Boccaccio, a former employee of the Foundation Archives, used materials still unavailable to other scholars at the time to write a brief, well-balanced summary of the Commission's activities: "Ground Itch and Dew Poison: The Rockefeller Sanitary Commission, 1909-14," *Journal of the History of Medicine and Allied Sciences,* 27 (January 1972), 30-53. James H. Cassedy drew on Stiles's articles, the published sources, and his own research into Stiles's efforts to counteract the German boycott of American pork, to write "The 'Germ of Laziness' in the South, 1900-1915: Charles Wardell Stiles and the Progressive Paradox," *Bulletin of the History of Medicine,* 45 (March-April 1971), 159-169. Cassedy argues that Stiles and his professional associates in the anti-hookworm campaign, although conservative and tradition-minded by training and inclination, "were still among the activists of their day in their willingness to extend statism in order to achieve social improvement" (pp. 168-169). Finally, Allen Tullos has written a fine article entitled "The Great Hookworm Crusade," in *Southern Exposure,* 6 (Summer 1978), 40-49.

Two more ambitious studies in the last few years have discussed the Sanitary Commission in the context of their larger purpose—to analyze the relationship between the growth and acceptance of scientific medicine and the American economic system. E. Richard Brown's *Rockefeller Medicine Men: Medicine and Capitalism in America* (Berkeley: University of California Press, 1979) is an outgrowth of his doctoral dissertation ("Physicians and Foundations: The Early Rockefeller Medical Philanthropies, 1900-1925," University of California at Berkeley, 1975). Howard S. Berliner has taken up much the same theme in "Philanthropic Foundations and Scientific Medicine," Sc.D. dissertation, The Johns Hopkins University, 1977. The points of view expressed in both studies are remarkably similar. Brown and Berliner see the Rockefellers' and Gates's philanthropic programs as functions of their class perspectives and hold them responsible, in large part, for the present state of American scientific research and health care. Harry Frank Farmer's "The Hookworm Program in the South, 1900-1925," Ph.D. dissertation, University of Georgia, 1970, also covers the decades before and after the Sanitary Commission and was written from published sources before the archival materials were opened to researchers. Farmer squarely places the anti-hookworm campaign in the vanguard of medical and social improvements that, in his view, have brought the South back from the dark days after the Civil War.

# Index